Nature's Way Handbook of Skin Care

Nature's Way Handbook of Skin Care

by

John Woodruff

Published on behalf of

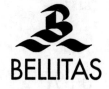

BELLITAS

by

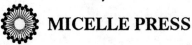

MICELLE PRESS

Weymouth, Dorset, England and Cranford, New Jersey, USA

British Library Cataloguing in Publication Data

Woodruff, John
    Nature's Way Handbook of Skin Care
    I. Title
    646.7
    ISBN 1-87022808-1

The information given in this book is presented in good faith but no warranty,
express or implied, is given nor can responsibility be accepted for problems
arising through the use or misuse of any Nature's Way product. All the
applications described are for the guidance of qualified beauty therapists who
are expected to use their professional judgement.

Bellitas Limited
Unit 12, Prospect Drive, Britannia Enterprise Park, Lichfield, Staffordshire,
WS14 9UX, England
Telephone (0543) 416611; Facsimile (0543) 416614

Micelle Press
12 Ullswater Crescent, Weymouth, Dorset DT3 5HE, England
Telephone and Facsimile (0305) 781574

Micelle Press, Inc.
P.O. Box 653, Cranford, NJ 07016, USA

Printed and bound in Great Britain by Dotesios Limited, Trowbridge, Wiltshire

Author's Note

When Bellitas asked me to write the *Nature's Way Handbook of Skin Care* to celebrate ten years of Nature's Way I was honoured to accept.

Seldom is a cosmetic chemist fortunate enough to be granted the freedom to create an entire skin-care range using the best materials available. I was able to do just that when Nature's Way was first conceived in 1982, and have been closely associated with the products ever since.

There have been many changes but the initial concept has remained unaltered — to provide high-quality, cruelty-free and cost-effective products for the beauty therapist that are fully tested for efficacy in use and long-term shelf-life.

Nature's Way has only ever been sold for professional use and throughout its history we have listened to the professional. We have tested every product in selected salons and colleges before releasing it for sale.

We have welcomed praise but listened to criticism and made changes where necessary. We acknowledge with grateful thanks the assistance provided by all those therapists who, over the years, have contributed their knowledge and ideas and have thus helped to make Nature's Way the leading range of skin-care products available to the professional in Britain.

Nature's Way is a dynamic range, always at the forefront of current thinking and responding to changing requirements. Thus Nature's Way Aromatherapy was introduced in 1991 and Sun Protect with UV-A and UV-B protection will be introduced with the publication of this book. The use of organosilanes in anticellulite therapy and the limiting of free radicals in ageing skin are also newly introduced to the Nature's Way range. Finally, the packaging itself has undergone change to reflect better the products' natural origins.

I gratefully acknowledge permission to reprint sections of certain articles which originally appeared in *Health & Beauty Salon* magazine and thank all those who helped and supported me through the writing of this book, especially Patricia Margret who made the drawings.

John Woodruff, Technical Consultant
56 Orchard Avenue
Lower Parkstone
Poole
Dorset BH14 8AJ

Telephone (0202) 741710; Facsimile (0202) 716007

Contents

Illustrations

Introduction

This step-by-step guide to the Nature's Way method of skin care is a unique handbook full of useful information for the busy beauty therapist.

It describes the common skin types and their disorders, it helps the therapist to select the best products for their treatment and gives a fully illustrated guide to their use.

It provides details on follow-up treatment at home, with tips on which products to sell to the client for home use, how to make that sale and how to keep the client satisfied and returning to the beauty therapist's salon to pay for the skills it provides.

The use of scrubs and masks is fully covered, and there is a section on galvanic treatment using Nature's Way ampoules.

A complete chapter is devoted to aromatherapy. The use of essential oils is covered in detail and an easy-to-use selection guide is an invaluable aid to effective salon treatment.

Every Nature's Way product is fully described, all its ingredients disclosed and the use of these materials in skin care is dealt with in detail. However, this book is more than a guide to Nature's Way products: it provides a complete description of the skin, its problems and the cosmetic means of alleviating them.

Here is an indispensable reference book which the beauty therapist will find a constant and valuable source of information.

Chapter One

The Skin

As a child, I thought the skin was simply an elastic envelope which held the body together and that without it we would ooze all over the place. However, I now know it to be the largest single organ of the human body with many other important functions. It has been described as a busy frontier which mediates between the organism and the environment.[1]

Skin not only controls the loss of vital fluids, but prevents the penetration of foreign substances, acts as a defence against the sun and cushions the body against mechanical shock. It transmits messages to the brain as a result of its sensitivity to stimuli. Skin is also important for heat control, allowing transmission of perspiration to cool the body down and contraction of blood vessels to conserve vital heat. With the eyes and hair, it is what people first see of us and a flawless complexion is the wish of all.

For those who like some facts and figures, here are a few interesting ones relating to the skin.

- The skin of an adult ranges in area from about 12,500 to 18,000 cm^2.
- It weighs about 3.2 kg in women and about 4.8 kg in men.
- Most of the skin has hair follicles with associated sebaceous glands and these number between 30 and 60 per cm^2 on the thighs, over 500 per cm^2 on the cheeks and over 800 per cm^2 on the forehead.[2]

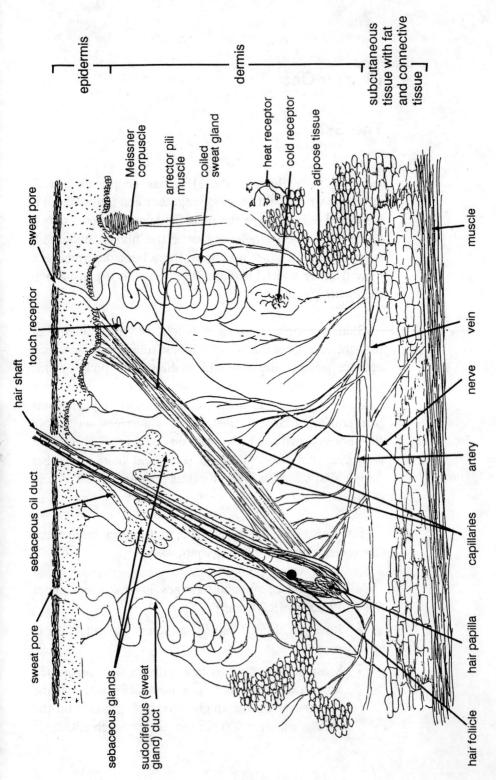

Figure 1. The skin (diagrammatic)

- The palms of the hands and soles of the feet have neither hair follicles nor sebaceous glands.
- One cm^2 of skin contains approximately 1.8 million cells and 37 cm of blood vessels.
- The skin contains about one million nerve fibres which terminate mostly on the face, hands and feet.
- The average thickness of the skin varies from 0.005 mm on the eyelids to 0.50 mm on the soles of the feet; over most of the body's surface it is between 0.01 and 0.02 mm in thickness.

There are three major recognisable regions of the skin: the epidermis, the dermis and the subcutaneous.

The skin's impermeability is due principally to the outer horny layer of the epidermis; if this is removed, the dermis is relatively permeable. The epidermis consists of two distinct layers separated by an intermediate zone. The outer layer is keratin arranged in strata known as epithelial tissue. It has no blood vessels, is free from pain nerve endings but is sensitive to touch. The outermost cells are dead scales which loosen and are shed. If they are not lost they appear as whitened dry cells and a powdery film. The correct name for the outer layer is *stratum corneum.*

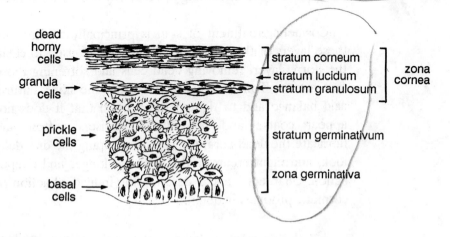

Figure 2. Detailed structure of the epidermis

The horny layer is readily dried through environmental factors — wind, sun, heat and cold — and when the skin is frequently subjected to such conditions the layer will thicken and may appear dry and flaky.

Below the outer layer of dead cells is the granular layer. It consists of cells in the process of keratinisation. The outer part of each cell becomes keratinised by an enzymatic process, the cell nuclei are digested and as the cell migrates towards the horny layer it becomes flattened. This layer is correctly termed the *stratum granulosum* and between it and the stratum corneum is a third stratum known as the *stratum lucidum*, which is a narrow translucent layer of eleidin.

The lower, or basal layer, is a zone of cell growth, starting with columns of cells arranged perpendicularly to the skin's surface. These gradually migrate towards the outer layer and as they separate from neighbouring cells they change shape, becoming elongated. They remain joined to other cells with fine threads filled with protoplasm, which give them their characteristic prickly appearance and hence their name of prickle cells. The average life cycle of each new cell from reproduction in the basal layer to discarding in the horny layer is six weeks.

Cosmetic treatment of skin is principally confined to these layers of the epidermis. Cleansers are used to clean the horny layer, removing dead cells and softening those that remain. Toners are used to restore the skin's natural acid balance and to tighten the skin so that it does not appear coarse and porous. Moisturisers soften and lubricate the dead keratinised cells, stopping the dry, flaky look, and night creams are left on for longer and deeper action. Chapters 2 and 3 describe the individual action of cosmetic products in detail.

The dermis is rich in blood vessels and contains the hair follicles, the sweat and sebaceous glands as well as the sensory nerve endings, all embedded in a network of elastic collagen fibrils. With ageing, this elasticity is lost, collagen is replaced with fatty globules and less water is held in the dermis, giving rise to wrinkles and dryness. The epidermis is a barrier between cosmetic products and the dermis, but hydrating masks, galvanic treatments and other products can have a beneficial action.

The subcutaneous region consists of yellow elastic fibres and white fibrous connective tissue. It is elastic and flexible and contains much fatty tissue. It allows the skin to move freely over the underlying muscular tissue and the fatty layer prevents excessive heat loss. This layer is thicker in women than men. The subcutaneous region is beyond the reach of most cosmetics, but massage and aromatherapy can be beneficial.

In the next chapter the cosmetic care of skin is described with particular reference to Nature's Way products.

Chapter Two

The Cosmetic Care of Skin

In an ideal world the visible areas of skin would be as flawless as those areas we normally keep clothed. Unfortunately, the action of sunlight, exposure to drying winds, to heat and to cold all combine to spoil this ideal. Add to this the mobility of the facial muscles which constantly stress and relax their protective covering, giving rise to laughter lines, character lines and wrinkles. We can then appreciate what therapeutic measures are necessary to restore those youthful good looks. But were they so good? Youthful skin may not have suffered environmental challenges for so long, but it has its own problems. From the eczema common in babies to teenage spots, youth is no guarantee of perfection.

What about post-youth to pre-middle age? This is the time when maintaining the skin in its optimum condition is so important if it is to remain at its best. Prophylactic treatment now will delay the onset of the next stage. As individuals age, their skin gradually becomes drier and loses its bloom and elasticity until eventually it becomes dehydrated, old and wrinkled.

Is this process inevitable? We cannot stop the ageing process but we can make it kinder. A friend says she likes a face to look as if it's been lived in and no one expects unlined perfection in latter middle age. However, a careful regime of skin care with professional advice and treatment can be amazingly beneficial.

The four essentials of cosmetic skin care are to *cleanse, tone, moisturise* and *replenish*.

A cleanser is normally a liquid emulsion which is used to remove facial grime. Normal bar soaps are generally thought to be too harsh, alkaline and drying for use on delicate facial tissues. Cleansers work by either emulsification or solvent action or both.

Most facial contamination is oily, either from make-up or sebum combined with perspiration and atmospheric pollution. These oily residues can be emulsified by the use of a very mild soap such as triethanolamine stearate. Alternatively, some cosmetic oils have very good solvent powers and will dissolve facial grease. In either case, once the grime has been loosened it can be removed with damp cotton wool along with all traces of excess product.

Technique for using a cleansing lotion:

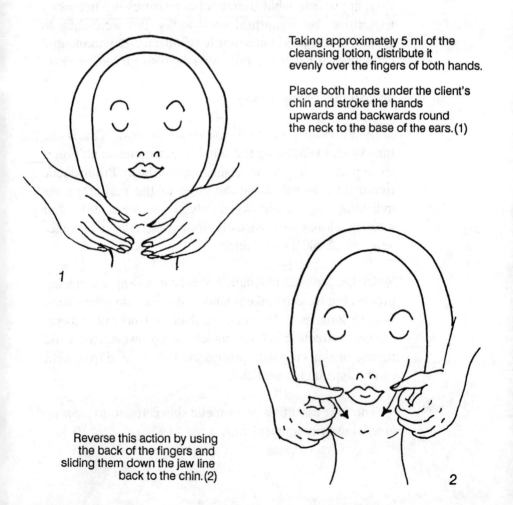

Taking approximately 5 ml of the cleansing lotion, distribute it evenly over the fingers of both hands.

Place both hands under the client's chin and stroke the hands upwards and backwards round the neck to the base of the ears. (1)

1

Reverse this action by using the back of the fingers and sliding them down the jaw line back to the chin. (2)

2

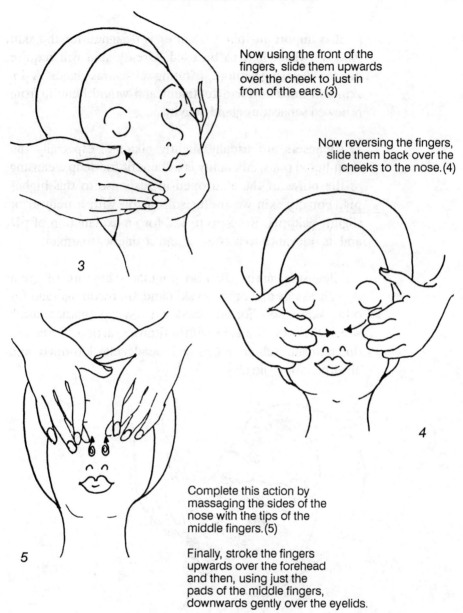

Now using the front of the fingers, slide them upwards over the cheek to just in front of the ears. (3)

Now reversing the fingers, slide them back over the cheeks to the nose. (4)

Complete this action by massaging the sides of the nose with the tips of the middle fingers. (5)

Finally, stroke the fingers upwards over the forehead and then, using just the pads of the middle fingers, downwards gently over the eyelids.

This forward and back action is repeated several times until the face is thoroughly covered with the product. It can then be removed with tissue, cotton wool or damp sponges depending on the nature of the product and the therapist's personal preferences.

The same technique may be used for applying creamy masks, facial massage creams, moisturisers and night cream.

Figure 3. Technique for using a cleansing lotion

It is important that a cleanser is designed for the skin type on which it is to be used. Greasy skin will require deeper cleansing without irritating sebaceous glands. A dry skin will need surface treatment and would benefit from renewed sebaceous gland activity.

Cleansers are usually slightly alkaline, especially the soap-based ones. Alkalinity is of benefit for deep cleansing as the pores of the skin open in response to this higher pH. For dry skin we prefer solvent oil with a neutral or slightly acid pH. Refer to p. 122 for an explanation of pH and its relevance to cosmetics and cosmetic treatment.

Cleansing masks are also popular. They are of great benefit to oily and problem skin and are recommended for other skin types. For an oily skin a clay-type mask is used, which dries on the skin with a drawing action. Pores are opened and sebum plugs and dead cells loosened and absorbed onto the clay.

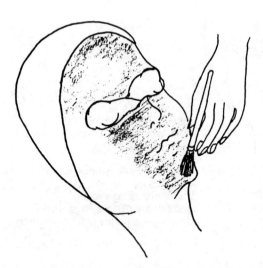

Figure 4. Application of a drying mask

As skin becomes drier, a different action is required, and oils and waxes are therefore incorporated into the product to prevent drying of the skin. The pH of masks for the drier skin is neutral or slightly acidic, and they have a stimulating and moisturising action rather than a cleansing and calming one.

Another way of cleansing the skin is to use a wash-off gel. The two available under the Nature's Way label are based on very mild surfactants; their action is deep cleansing without being drying. For oily skin, a special facial wash with bactericidal action has been developed and is used as a precursor to the mask.

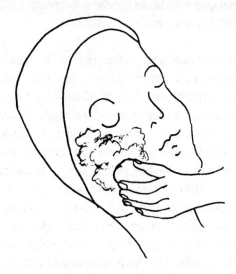

Figure 5. Use of facial wash and wash-off gels

After cleansing, the skin feels slightly oily, open-pored and vulnerable. A good quality toner will remove surface oils, close pores and leave the skin feeling refreshed, soothed and silky smooth. Cleansers are usually slightly alkaline: by incorporating a pH adjuster in the toner the skin's natural acid mantle is rapidly restored. This natural acidity is a barrier to bacteriological infection, and normal skin functions are also at their optimum at this pH.

All Nature's Way skin toners have two common ingredients, sodium lactate and witch hazel. Sodium lactate is a normal ingredient of skin perspiration; it is responsible for the pH of the acid mantle and has moisturising properties. Witch hazel is an essential constituent of all good skin toners. It is mildly astringent, soothing and healing.

Normally the product base is an aqueous-alcoholic lotion. The alcohol is present to confer mild astringency to the product and to make it cooling and refreshing with antiseptic qualities. Its concentration is varied according to the skin type for which the product is designed. A greasy skin needs more astringency, a dry skin very little. Because some people may be sensitive to alcohol it is not present in the Aloe Vera toner.

When clean and refreshed with toner, skin needs protection and replenishment of lost natural oils and moisture regulators. Two products are available in almost every range, a moisturiser and a night cream. The former is generally a soft emulsion which is easily applied and quickly dries to a matt finish. The latter is an oilier product which is more suitable for leaving overnight. However, in harsh conditions, cold winter winds, hot dry weather, or when involved in outdoor leisure activities, the use of a night cream is often beneficial during the daytime. Moisturisers are normally oil-in-water emulsions: they contain ingredients which hold water and their constituent oils are light, easily spread and dry readily to give a good base for make-up.

Moisturisers and night creams remain on the skin for extended periods, giving more time for active ingredients to transmit their benefits, but care has to be taken to ensure that they are of sufficient concentration to be effective and the base must be safe to use over a long period.

Night creams are of high oil content: they do not dry quickly but stay oily long enough to be massaged for a period, this massaging action being very beneficial to the facial tissues. Night creams for drier skins have penetrating vegetable oils which will slowly be absorbed into the skin's outer layers during the night. Mineral oils are sometimes used for their lubricity to assist in the massage action. Essential ingredients are usually at their highest concentration in night cream.

As we go from creams for normal skin to those for dry skin, the oil content of the emulsion is increased, and lighter, quickly absorbing oils are replaced with more penetrating and slower drying ones. An oily film on the face will retard transepidermal water loss and the water content of the cells will increase. This is very beneficial in skin that is losing its natural elasticity through collagen decay.

Night creams, as their name implies, are used at night. For salon treatment of dry skin and for weekly use at home, an application of a hydrating mask can make an immediate visible improvement. Hydrating masks are applied for between 10 and 15 minutes to cleansed skin. They usually contain metabolic stimulating agents to increase cellular activity whilst at the same time an occlusive film prevents water loss. The epidermis is softened and made more supple whilst the underlying layers are engorged with moisture, making them firm and more elastic. Whilst the effects gradually decrease with time, a supporting programme of daytime moisturising and night-time replenishment will help stabilise the visible improvement.

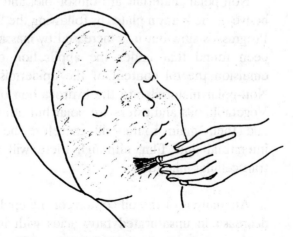

Figure 6. Application of a hydrating mask

Many people regard the skin as a plastic raincoat, impervious to all outside substances. Whilst its barrier properties are an important function, it is by no means impermeable to all materials. There are two main routes through the epidermis, the intercellular route and the transcellular. The stratum corneum consists of plates of keratin in a film of oil. Keratin can absorb water and swell, and this action opens the structure of the epidermis allowing polar substances, which are soluble in water, to pass through the cell using the water molecules as a pathway. Common polar cosmetic ingredients are propylene glycol, much used as a moisturiser, many surfactants, plant extracts and the volatile fractions of essential oils.

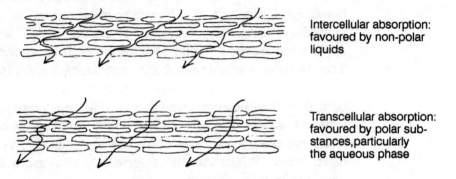

Intercellular absorption: favoured by non-polar liquids

Transcellular absorption: favoured by polar substances, particularly the aqueous phase

Figure 7. Percutaneous absorption

Non-polar materials are oil-soluble, and they progress between the keratin plates by following the lipid pathways. Progress is slow but it is increased by massage, and it has been found that under the application of a cosmetic emulsion the oil content of the epidermis is increased. Non-polar materials are the hydrocarbon oils and waxes. Vegetable oils and esters are polar but not water-soluble, and their main route will therefore be through the interstitial lipid film, although there will also be some transcellular migration.

An analysis of the oil content of the epidermis shows a decrease in unsaturated fatty acids with increasing age.

These materials are present in many vegetable oils and may explain why they are more effective in combating dry skin than mineral oil.

Two words in skin-care products are often confused: absorption and adsorption. If a material enters the cells it is absorbed; if it forms a substantive film over the surface it is adsorbed.

Absorption: favoured by polar materials and cellular structures

Adsorption: favoured by rough surfaces and substantive materials, e.g. proteins, oils and cationic substances

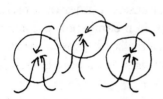
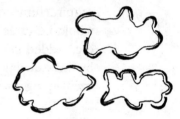

Figure 8. Absorption and adsorption

Absorbed materials actually enter the epidermis and may penetrate to the dermis; some even enter the blood stream. Adsorbed materials can form protective films on the epidermis and give the skin a smooth and pleasant feel. One such material is protein, whether of animal or vegetable origin. Its molecules are too large to enter the skin cells but it has a strong affinity for skin and will hold moisture to it. Interestingly, the rougher the surface, the greater the adsorption between the substrate and the adsorbing material, a phenomenon made much use of in protein hair treatments.

Too many cosmetic products reach the market place with very little thought as to their intended function and how their constituent ingredients are going to fulfil that function. One sees products for greasy skin which contain recognised comedone-forming materials; products for mature skin which contain ingredients with a drying action; products in which the pH and its likely effect on the natural acid mantle have been completely disregarded. Materials that are phototoxic are used in facial products and plant extracts are incorporated in minute quantities to make a pretty label rather than to utilise their benefits, the knowledge of which has been passed down through generations.

When formulating Nature's Way products, the different skin types with their associated problems were first identified. An ingredient which would be of particular benefit for each skin type was then specified and the range designed around that material. The functional requirements of each product were studied so that it would be effective as a cleanser, a toner or a moisturiser, etc. Added benefits were then conferred to each product by introducing herbal extracts of proven worth or by exchanging one oily component for a more beneficial one.

Throughout the formulation stage natural materials or materials based on natural vegetable products were used wherever practical. We are very aware that many people find using animal products disagreeable, and no materials known to be of animal origin are used in any of the Nature's Way ranges. Collagen is usually of animal origin but Nature's Way uses a special one of vegetable extraction. Refer to p. 53 for more information on this material.

Although natural ingredients are used as much as possible, preservatives have to be included or the products would rapidly deteriorate. In most products a little fragrance is incorporated and some are tinted to enhance their appeal. No Nature's Way product has ever been tested on animals, nor have any of the ingredients been animal-tested on behalf of Nature's Way. The materials used have established their safety through long-term use, and Nature's Way can therefore categorically state:

> **> Never Tested on Animals <**

In the next chapter we will look at some common skin types and the products available to care for them. The products are fully described and the principal ingredients mentioned. In chapter 9 will be found a full ingredient listing of all Nature's Way products and chapter 3 describes the function of these materials in cosmetic skin care.

Chapter Three

Skin Types, Their Recognition and Cosmetic Treatment

A step-by-step guide to a treatment programme

- Identify skin type
- Identify problems
- Select optimum group of products
- Cleanse, tone, moisturise, replenish
- Post-treatment and continuation at home

Some skin types are immediately obvious — the greasy skin of youth, the dry skin of the elderly. Other skins are a combination of oily and normal or normal-to-dry. Many clients may not know what their skin type is, but most will think it delicate and in need of special care. Nature's Way ranges of products have been carefully designed to cater for all skin types. Please remember, though, that there is no sharp division between each skin type and each product range and that there is a choice of two ranges for almost any type of skin.

In the following pages we first identify skin types and their related problems and the cause of these problems, and then look at means of cosmetic treatment.

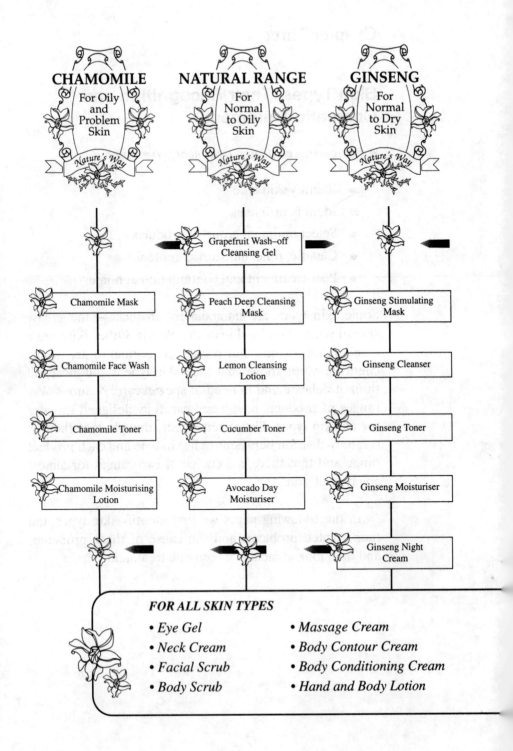

CHAMOMILE
For Oily
and
Problem
Skin

NATURAL RANGE
For
Normal
to Oily
Skin

GINSENG
For
Normal
to Dry
Skin

Grapefruit Wash–off
Cleansing Gel

Chamomile Mask	Peach Deep Cleansing Mask	Ginseng Stimulating Mask
Chamomile Face Wash	Lemon Cleansing Lotion	Ginseng Cleanser
Chamomile Toner	Cucumber Toner	Ginseng Toner
Chamomile Moisturising Lotion	Avocado Day Moisturiser	Ginseng Moisturiser
		Ginseng Night Cream

FOR ALL SKIN TYPES
- *Eye Gel*
- *Neck Cream*
- *Facial Scrub*
- *Body Scrub*
- *Massage Cream*
- *Body Contour Cream*
- *Body Conditioning Cream*
- *Hand and Body Lotion*

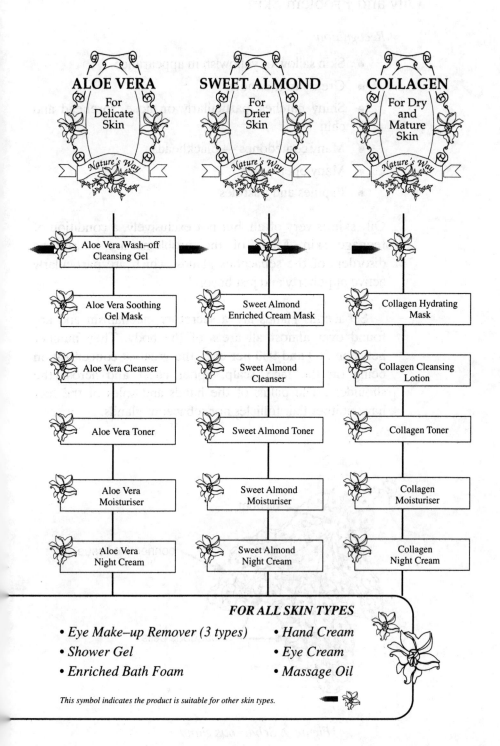

ALOE VERA
For Delicate Skin
Nature's Way

SWEET ALMOND
For Drier Skin
Nature's Way

COLLAGEN
For Dry and Mature Skin
Nature's Way

Aloe Vera Wash–off Cleansing Gel

Aloe Vera Soothing Gel Mask	Sweet Almond Enriched Cream Mask	Collagen Hydrating Mask
Aloe Vera Cleanser	Sweet Almond Cleanser	Collagen Cleansing Lotion
Aloe Vera Toner	Sweet Almond Toner	Collagen Toner
Aloe Vera Moisturiser	Sweet Almond Moisturiser	Collagen Moisturiser
Aloe Vera Night Cream	Sweet Almond Night Cream	Collagen Night Cream

FOR ALL SKIN TYPES

• *Eye Make–up Remover (3 types)*
• *Shower Gel*
• *Enriched Bath Foam*

• *Hand Cream*
• *Eye Cream*
• *Massage Oil*

This symbol indicates the product is suitable for other skin types.

Oily and Problem Skin

Recognition

- Skin sallow or yellowish in appearance
- Greasy to the touch
- Shiny patches, particularly on nose, forehead and chin
- Many comedones — blackheads
- Many open pores
- Papules and pustules

Oily skin is very often, but not exclusively, a condition of teenage skin. Many of the problems are caused by disorders of the sebaceous glands, which are particularly active at puberty and just beyond.

Sebaceous glands are a secretory mechanism and are found over almost all areas of the body. They number between 500 and 900 per cm^2, the greatest concentration being on the face, scalp, upper chest and across the shoulders. The palms of the hands and soles of the feet have neither hair follicles nor sebaceous glands.

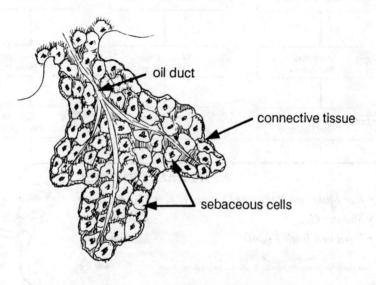

Figure 9. Sebaceous gland

Sebaceous glands secrete sebum, which is an oily mixture of glycerides, free fatty acids, wax esters, squalane and cholesterol. The function of sebum is uncertain: it has some antifungal activity and is believed to contain pheromones, which are excretions of sexually attractive odours, much used in the animal kingdom but obscured by washing and perfume application in humans. A third function, as yet unproven, is that seborrhoea may boost the skin's natural immune system.

Sebaceous gland activity is minimal in children but at puberty it may increase fivefold. Sebaceous glands are stimulated by the male hormone androgen found in the andrenal cortex and in women androgen is also secreted by the ovaries.

Sebaceous glands do not constantly exude their oil. Within the gland cells grow, accumulating lipid, swelling the gland to several times its original size. It then disintegrates releasing its contents before the process starts all over again. Such a process is termed holacrine.

Sebaceous gland activity is subject to problems which lead to the papules and pustules of *Acne vulgaris*. The most common cause is hyperkeratinisation at the neck of the follicle. Excessive keratin blocks the exit of sebum from the gland and the build-up of sebum eventually ruptures into the dermis. Bacterial infection then occurs and the familiar pimples of acne manifest themselves on the sufferer's face.

In summary, therefore, the process is:

- High level of sebaceous gland activity
- Hyperkeratinisation leading to blocked pores and comedones
- Sebum build-up
- Rupture into the dermis
- Bacterial infection
- Pimples

The cosmetic treatment of acne must be to keep the skin clean and free from blocked pores and to avoid bacterial infection. Products must not stimulate further sebaceous gland activity by irritation and must avoid the formation of comedones at all costs. The cause is a combination of factors, the alleviation of which must also be a combination of treatments.

Remember that one treatment is never going to correct a situation that may have been building up for months. Young people are not going to come for treatment until they have tried many things themselves, some good, some bad. Frequently all else has failed and now they are turning to you for an instant, miracle cure.

The first consultation should be more talk than action. Make the client comfortable, ask about life-style, diet, drinking, smoking, exercise. Treat the whole person: you are projecting your image as a caring person who has the client's best interests at heart, but you must be genuine and sincere.

Explain the cause and effect of the problem and what you are going to do about it. Explain that it takes time and effort by both of you and that the home treatment and advice on diet and life-style are as important as the professional treatment by yourself.

If you are successful, the client's friends will be shortly making appointments, and before long you will be the local expert. Also, a client at this age could be a client for life as skin care does not stop with the ending of acne.

Nature's Way approach is the Chamomile range which has been specifically designed to treat oily and problem skin and is based on a regime of gentle cleaning, soothing and protection. Care has been taken to exclude from the range all known comedonic materials, such as free fatty acids and fatty acid esters.

Nature's Way Chamomile range is not only for skins showing visible signs of acne: we believe in treating the underlying cause, which is a high level of sebaceous gland activity associated with blocked pores and bacterial infection; and, as always, prevention is better than cure.

The bacteria, *Acne bacillus*, exist in vast numbers in the sebaceous glands and it is their infection which causes comedones by breaking down the sebum into free fatty acids. These bind keratin scales together and a mixture of dead keratin, bacteria and sebum forms a black plug at the exit of the hair follicle.

The first stage is to cleanse deeply the face and other problem areas, which may include the upper chest and shoulders.

1. Remove all make-up, first with tissue, then with Chamomile Face Wash, taking care not to break any skin over the pustules. This should be done by rinsing the face and then applying the Face Wash on damp cotton wool or with a soft facial brush. Use small circular motions all over the face and neck, working up a soft cleansing foam. Rinse well with warm water and pat the area dry with a clean tissue.

Examine the skin. If there are signs of comedones or blocked pores or other indications of impurities within the skin, Chamomile Mask should now be used.

Apply a thin layer with a mask brush to the face, leave for 10 to 15 minutes, then remove with damp sponges.

2. Depending on the severity of the problem, either wipe off all remaining traces of the mask with tissue dampened with Chamomile Toner or repeat Step 1 with Chamomile Face Wash and then apply Chamomile Toner.

3. Finally, apply Chamomile Moisturiser Lotion, which is a non-oily preparation, to soothe and protect the skin. It

should be applied on cotton wool to all the treated areas. Do not apply make-up or camouflage creams and ask the client to keep their use to a minimum. The client will be self-conscious about her problems: explain that bright lips and eyes will draw attention away from a flawed complexion.

Treatment summary

Salon treatment

1. Cleanse using mildly medicated Chamomile Face Wash and Chamomile Face Mask.

2. Tone with Nature's Way Chamomile Toner.

3. Protect with Chamomile Moisturiser Lotion.

4. If make-up is required, use cake or water-based foundation.

Home care

Daily:

1. Remove make-up and cleanse with Nature's Way mildly medicated Chamomile Face Wash.

2. Tone with Nature's Way Chamomile Toner.

3. Moisturise lightly with Nature's Way Chamomile Moisturiser Lotion.

Twice weekly:

1. Face mask — thinly apply Nature's Way Chamomile Mask.

2. Steam — fill a bowl with hot water and add a tablespoon of Nature's Way Aromatherapy Oil of Lavender or Rosemary. Place a towel over the head and bend face over steam for 3 minutes, rinse the face with warm water and tone as usual.

Do's: Pay particular attention to diet, avoiding very greasy or sugary foods such as chips, chocolates and fizzy drinks. Try to eat more fresh fruit and vegetables.

Don'ts: Never pick or squeeze spots as this may cause permanent scarring and spreading of infection.

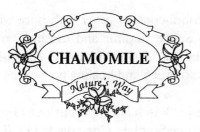 for Oily and Problem Skin

Chamomile Face Wash

Toilet soap is usually very alkaline and can irritate the sebaceous glands, thereby stimulating more sebum production. This can be avoided by using a carefully designed liquid face wash. Nature's Way Chamomile Face Wash uses mild surfactants, thickened with an ethoxylated ester, and contains the bactericide propylene phenoxytol. Its pH is 5.3 so that it does not affect the natural acid balance of the skin and it contains pure essential oil of chamomile, renowned for its soothing and healing properties.

Principal ingredients: Propylene Phenoxytol, Lauryl Betaine, Sodium Laureth Sulphate, PEG-150 Distearate, Chamomile Oil.

Chamomile Mask

A deep cleaning, non-oily mask that softens the blockages in the pores and, by its drawing action, absorbs the comedones and sebum. In common with the other Chamomile products, it also contains essential oil of chamomile and the pH is adjusted to 5.3 using sodium lactate.

Principal ingredients: Chamomile Oil, Biological Sulphur, Propylene Glycol, Magnesium Aluminium Silicate, Kaolin.

Chamomile Toner

This is a low-alcohol-content toner with pure witch hazel plus biologically active sulphur and rosemary oil. Its pH has been adjusted to 5.3 and natural chamomile oil has been used for its soothing and healing properties.

Principal ingredients: Witch Hazel, Propylene Glycol, Rosemary Oil, Active Sulphur, Chamomile Oil, Ethanol, Sodium Lactate.

Chamomile Moisturiser Lotion

This smooth, protective emulsion is based on natural oils and waxes, containing zinc oxide for its soothing properties and a very effective moisturising system based on the skin's natural moisturising factor (NMF). The product has been thickened with xanthan gum to give it body without stickiness and pigmented to blend into the skin. The product is pH balanced at 5.3 and contains essential oil of chamomile.

Principal ingredients: Zinc Oxide, Emulsifiers, Almond Oil, Cocoa Butter, Sodium Lactate, Xanthan Gum, Chamomile Oil.

Normal-to-Oily Skin

Recognition

Obviously not so oily as the problem skin associated with seborrhoea, but still with an oily sheen across the forehead and down the central panel. In general such a skin is in good condition and the client can be satisfied that oily skin visibly ages more slowly than dry skin. Treatment should concentrate on keeping the skin clean and well toned. Oily areas may still be subject to comedones and some acne formation, whereas the cheeks may need a light moisturiser.

Nature's Way treatment programme for oily-to-normal skin is to use the Natural range with its deep-acting Peach Deep Cleansing Mask to ensure maximum cleansing and a choice of cleansers to suit all clients. Cucumber Toner maintains the skin's natural acid balance and Avocado Day Moisturiser restores its bloom without oiliness.

Salon treatment

1. Remove all make-up, first with tissue, then by using Grapefruit Wash-off Cleansing Gel by rinsing the face and then applying the Wash-off Cleanser on damp cotton wool or with a soft facial brush. Use small circular motions all over the face and neck, working up a soft cleansing foam. Rinse well with warm water and pat area dry with clean tissue.

2. Examine the skin. If there are signs of comedones or blocked pores or other indications of impurities within the skin, Peach Deep Cleansing Mask should now be used.

Apply a thin layer with a mask brush to the face, leave for 10 to 15 minutes, then remove with damp sponges.

3. Wipe off all remaining traces of the mask with tissue dampened with Cucumber Toner.

4. Moisturise using light and creamy Nature's Way Avocado Day Moisturiser, paying particular attention to the drier areas of cheeks and throat.

5. Foundation: a water-based fluid make-up with no-shine powder on nose, forehead and chin is recommended.

Alternative treatment

If the skin shows little sign of oiliness, use Lemon Cleansing Lotion for the cleaning stage followed by Cucumber Toner and Avocado Day Moisturiser.

Home care

Daily:

1. Cleanse using either Nature's Way Grapefruit Wash-off Cleansing Gel or Lemon Cleansing Lotion, as preferred.

2. Tone with Nature's Way Cucumber Skin Tonic.

3. Moisturise with Nature's Way Avocado Day Moisturiser on all areas.

Weekly:

1. Apply Peach Deep Cleansing Mask

2. Steam — as for greasy skin if not too many dilated arterioles on cheeks. For combination skin, elder flowers or horsetail herbs may be added to the water.

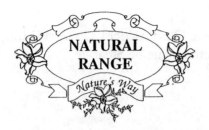

for Normal-to-Oily Skin

Peach Deep Cleansing Mask

A deep cleansing mask specifically designed for oily-to-normal skin. Its penetrating action softens the keratin and sebum that block pores and cause comedones and as it dries it draws these impurities out of the skin.

Principal ingredients: Magnesium Aluminium Silicate, Zinc Oxide, Xanthan Gum, Propylene Glycol, Beeswax, Peach Kernel Oil.

Grapefruit Wash-off Cleansing Gel

A refreshing alternative to harsh alkaline soaps for facial cleansing. The principal constituent has a truly frightful name behind which is hiding one of the mildest cleansing agents available for skin cleansing. With the addition of grapefruit juice and thickened with a skin-friendly distearate that leaves the skin feeling silky smooth, this is a superb product. Please do not expect masses of bubbles — they usually mean harsh detergents; Grapefruit Wash-off Cleansing Gel will just give a soft gentle foam.

Principal ingredients: Cocoamphocarboxyglycinate, Grapefruit Juice, PEG-150 Distearate.

Lemon Cleansing Lotion

This cleansing lotion is of the mild liquid-soap type based on triethanolamine stearate with oleyl alcohol for deep cleaning penetration. It is slightly alkaline so that pores are opened and impurities emulsified away. It contains pure lemon juice.

Principal ingredients: Oleyl Alcohol, Glyceryl Esters, Pure Lemon Juice, Triethanolamine Stearate.

Cucumber Toner

A refreshing, mildly astringent skin toner based on glycerine, witch hazel and ethanol. The pH is adjusted to 5.3 with lactic acid and the product contains natural extract of cucumber.

Principal ingredients: Glycerine, Witch Hazel, Cucumber Extract, Ethanol, Lactic Acid, Sodium Lactate.

Avocado Day Moisturiser

This is a natural moisturising cream for normal and combination skin. It contains cocoa butter, almond oil and avocado oil for emollience and glycerine and sodium lactate for moisture control. It can be used under make-up and be used at night if dry patches develop, perhaps because of exposure to drying winds.

Principal ingredients: Avocado Oil, Emulsifiers, Sweet Almond Oil, Cocoa Butter, Glycerine, Sodium Lactate.

Normal-to-Dry Skin

No products for normal skin? If by "normal" we mean perfect, then no skin ever appears to be truly normal. The Natural range caters for the normal-tending-to-oily skin, the Ginseng range for normal-tending-towards-dry. Please remember the overlap each product range has and experiment to find the perfect ones for your needs.

Recognition

Although the skin is in general good health, it may have dry, flaky patches, particularly on the cheeks. The throat may also be showing signs of early wrinkling. Cheeks tend to be particularly dry and often have dilated arterioles and milia.

Salon treatment

1. Remove all make-up, first with tissue, then you may wish to use either Grapefruit or Aloe Vera Wash-off Cleansing Gel. Rinse the face, then apply the Wash-off Cleanser on damp cotton wool or with a soft facial brush. Work up a soft cleansing foam with small circular movements, rinse well with warm water and pat the area dry with clean tissue.

2. Examine the skin and decide whether to use a face mask or cleansing lotion for the next stage. If treatment is taking place in a salon this decision may depend on the time available and the client's wishes.

3a. Ginseng Stimulating Mask is ideal for this skin type; apply a thin layer with a mask brush to the face and neck, leave for 10 to 15 minutes and then remove with cotton wool or tissue.

3b. Alternatively, use Nature's Way Ginseng Cleanser, apply to face and neck, massage gently into the skin to emulsify sebum and loosen dead keratin, then remove with cotton wool.

4. When the skin is thoroughly cleansed, restore its natural pH balance by freshening the skin with Ginseng Toner and leave to dry naturally.

5. A light application of Ginseng Moisturiser completes the salon treatment. Massage it gently into the skin until fully absorbed; its light and non-greasy texture makes it ideal for use under make-up.

6. Eye Gel could be applied after facial treatments to soothe and restore the skin's natural equilibrium in the eye area.

7. At night apply Ginseng Night Cream to the face and neck, massage well with smooth, upright strokes, paying special attention to the throat and cheeks. On cold, winter days use Ginseng Night Cream for daytime protection.

Treatment summary

1. Remove make-up and examine skin.

2. Use Ginseng Mask or Cleanser.

3. Tone with Ginseng Toner.

4. Apply Ginseng Moisturiser.

5. At night use Ginseng Night Cream.

6. Additional products— Eye Gel.

Home care

Daily:

1. Remove make-up with Nature's Way Ginseng Cleanser or a Wash-off Gel.

2. Tone using mild Nature's Way Ginseng Toner on face and neck areas.

3. Moisturise — paying particular attention to cheeks and neck — with rich and creamy Nature's Way Ginseng Moisturiser.

4. At night stimulate the tissues and protect and rehydrate the skin by massaging Ginseng Night Cream into the face and neck.

Twice weekly:

1. Face mask — apply Ginseng Stimulating Mask liberally to the face and neck area using a clean spatula. Relax for 10 to 15 minutes, then remove the excess mask with clean tissue and apply Ginseng Toner followed by Moisturiser or Night Cream.

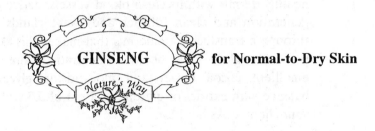

GINSENG   **for Normal-to-Dry Skin**

The Ginseng range of products is ideal for general-purpose use and is very popular with colleges. Each product contains extract of ginseng, a plant whose root, in particular, is valued by the Chinese in botanical medicine. Ancient Chinese medical texts claim it to be a tonic, a stimulant, a carminative (curing flatulence) and a demulcent (soothing agent). In traditional Chinese medicine it is quoted as:

> "a tonic to the five viscera, quieting animal spirits, establishing the opening up of the heart, benefiting the understanding and awakening and prolonging sexual potency."[3]

Interestingly, an almost identical plant was found by early settlers in Eastern America which was an essential part of Red Indian medicinal folklore and to which similar properties were attributed. The plant itself grows very slowly, taking about six years to become ready for harvest.

It has always been very expensive and is difficult to cultivate.

We cannot claim that Nature's Way Ginseng products will bestow all the benefits on the user that are claimed by the Chinese and North American Indians, but it is thought to stimulate epidermal metabolism, bringing extra vitality to the skin.

Ginseng Stimulating Face Mask

This light, non-greasy mask stimulates epidermal metabolism, restoring a natural bloom to the skin. It is a healthy dermis with its fresh blood vessels, active cellular generation and clean follicles and sweat glands shining through a translucent epidermis that makes this skin type positively glow with health. Penetrating almond oil, emollient cocoa butter and moisturising glycerine in balance with extract of ginseng at a pH of 5.3 will ensure your client looks her best.

Principal ingredients: Extract of Ginseng, Sodium Lactate, Glycerine, Sweet Almond Oil, Cocoa Butter.

Ginseng Cleanser

An effective cleanser suitable for normal-to-dry skin. It contains extract of ginseng, valued for the extra vitality it brings to the skin. It is essential when designing a cleanser for drier skin types that it does not leave the epidermis stripped of all its protective oils. With Ginseng Cleanser, Nature's Way has achieved this fine balance of cleansing without de-oiling.

Principal ingredients: Extract of Ginseng, Oleyl Alcohol, Glyceryl Esters, Triethanolamine Stearate, Cetearyl Alcohol.

Ginseng Toner

Ginseng Toner is mildly astringent, pH-balanced to match the skin's natural pH and contains witch hazel, an essential ingredient of all good skin toners. Extract of ginseng is included for its stimulating effects.

Principal ingredients: Extract of Ginseng, Ethanol, Sodium Lactate, Glycerine, Witch Hazel, Essential Oils.

Ginseng Moisturiser

For the normal-to-dry skin a light, readily applied moisturiser is required that will rehydrate drier areas without making the entire face feel oily. Ginseng Moisturiser achieves this by a careful combination of emollient oils, waxes and emulsifiers.

Principal ingredients: Extract of Ginseng, Glycerine, cosmetic oils and waxes principally from Palm Oil and all incorporated to give protection without greasiness.

Ginseng Night Cream

At night, skin that is starting to show dryness needs extra stimulation. By massaging Ginseng Night Cream into the facial tissues, this stimulation is achieved and the skin gains from all-night contact with its beneficial oils.

Principal ingredients: Extract of Ginseng, Borax, Cetearyl Alcohol, Propylene Glycol, Glyceryl Esters, Petrolatum.

Delicate Skin

Recognition

Delicate skin often tends towards dryness; it may also display the following characteristics:

- Many dilated arterioles
- Delicate to the touch
- Highly coloured — reddens easily
- Dry and flaky patches
- Small acid spots around the mouth
- Freckles over the face
- Pale complexion
- Prone to allergies

The Aloe Vera range has been developed specifically for skins having problems of sensitivity. The products are free of all known allergens and are designed to give protection against environmental harm from sunlight, drying atmospheres and allergic responses to atmospheric pollution.

Salon treatment

1. Remove all make-up, first with tissue, then you may wish to use Aloe Vera Wash-off Cleansing Gel. Rinse the face, then apply Aloe Vera Wash-off Cleansing Gel on damp cotton wool or with a soft facial brush. Work up a gentle foam and rinse with warm water and gently pat dry.

2. Examine the skin and decide whether to use a face mask or cleansing lotion for the next stage. If the treatment is taking place in a salon this decision may depend on the time available and the client's wishes.

3a. Aloe Vera Soothing Face Mask is ideal for this skin type. Apply a thin layer with a mask brush to the face and neck, leave for 10 to 15 minutes and then remove with cotton wool or tissue.

3b. Alternatively, use Nature's Way Aloe Vera Cleanser, apply to face and neck, massage gently into the skin to emulsify sebum and loosen dead keratin, then remove with cotton wool.

4. When the skin is thoroughly cleansed, restore its natural pH balance by freshening the skin with Aloe Vera Toner and gently blot dry.

5. A light application of Aloe Vera Moisturiser completes the salon treatment. Massage it gently into the skin until fully absorbed; its light and non-greasy texture makes it ideal for use under make-up.

6. Eye Gel could be applied after facial treatments to soothe and restore the skin's natural equilibrium in the eye area.

7. At night apply Aloe Vera Night Cream to the face and neck, massage well with smooth, upright strokes, paying special attention to the throat and cheeks. On cold, winter days use Aloe Vera Night Cream for daytime protection.

Home care

1. Cleanse, tone and moisturise as for salon treatment. The moisturiser contains ingredients to protect the skin from ultraviolet radiation and also contains film-forming ingredients which put a barrier between the skin and the environment. The moisturiser should always be applied before using make-up.

2. At night, replenish the skin's natural protection with Aloe Vera Night Cream gently massaged into all areas that are normally exposed to sunlight.

Do's: The protection of a delicate skin is of paramount importance, and particular attention should be given to any areas of dilated arterioles — red veins — or dry patches. Moisturise liberally, therefore, more than once a day if necessary.

Don'ts: Steaming and the use of soap may be positively harmful to this skin type if many dilated arterioles are present. Avoid over-drying or stimulating the skin, and always remember to blot the skin dry after toning.

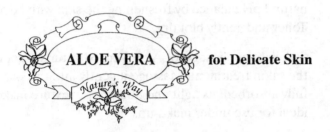

ALOE VERA   for Delicate Skin

Of all the ingredients chosen from nature for their claim to benefit human skin, the gel extracted from the aloe vera plant is perhaps the most interesting. Renowned for its healing properties, especially for skin damaged by burns or sensitive to other cosmetic ingredients, aloe vera gel is an essential ingredient of all Nature's Way products for delicate skin.

None of the aloe vera products contains mineral oil, ethyl alcohol or lanolin or any other cosmetic ingredient known to cause occasional allergic problems.

The only fragrance used is essential oil of chamomile, renowned for its skin-soothing properties, and the only colour used is azulene, the calming agent found only in natural chamomile oil. Although primarily for dry skin, the products are light enough for all skin types.

Aloe Vera Wash-off Cleansing Gel

A soothing alternative to harsh alkaline soaps for facial cleansing. The principal constituent has a truly frightful name behind which is hiding one of the mildest cleansing agents available for skin cleansing. With the addition of aloe vera gel and thickened with a skin-friendly distearate that leaves the skin feeling silky smooth, this is a superb product. Please do not expect masses of bubbles — they usually mean harsh detergents; Aloe Vera Wash-off Cleansing Gel will just give a soft gentle foam.

Principal ingredients: Cocoamphocarboxyglycinate, Aloe Vera Gel, PEG-150 Distearate.

Aloe Vera Soothing Gel Mask

This non-drying mask softens the outer layers of keratin, allowing its moisturisers to slowly penetrate the cells through transcellular migration. After 10 to 15 minutes, gentle removal with tissue will also remove any loose keratin and the arterioles will be soothed and calmed.

Principal ingredients: Aloe Vera Gel, Glycerine, Witch Hazel, Carbomer.

Aloe Vera Cleanser

Aloe Vera Gel blended with almond oil and other vegetable oils in a natural liquid-soap base. This product is designed to gently cleanse the skin, leaving it glowing with health and vitality while treating it with care and tenderness.

Principal ingredients: Aloe Vera Gel, Almond Oil, Caprylic/Capric Triglyceride, Triethanolamine Stearate, Glyceryl Esters, Polyglycerylmethacrylate.

Aloe Vera Toner

A non-alcoholic toning lotion which gives the skin a mild astringency after cleansing. It restores the natural pH of the acid mantle and imparts a soft, smooth after-feel.

Principal ingredients: Witch Hazel, Aloe Vera Gel, Azulene, Sodium Lactate, Propylene Glycol.

Aloe Vera Moisturiser

This unique Nature's Way product is a moisturiser which combines a richness of ingredients with ready absorption by the skin. It gives protection against UV-A and UV-B light and, by imparting a supple occlusive film to the skin, gives day-long moisturising. It is ideal for use under make-up and will protect against many potential allergens.

Principal ingredients: Aloe Vera Gel, Cocoa Butter, Almond Oil, Avocado Oil, Caprylic/Capric Triglyceride, Vegetable Beeswax, Silicone Oil, UV Light Screen, Chamomile Oil, Sodium Lactate.

Aloe Vera Night Cream

A night cream is the essential end to the day's skin-care routine. All skin types benefit from night-long replenishment of the skin's natural caring and protecting agents. Even oily skins gain from stimulating blood circulation by the massage of a little Aloe Vera Night Cream into the face and neck. This cream is so rich and yet readily absorbed that it is used by many people throughout the day, especially those engaged in outdoor sports such as sailing and skiing, and for this reason it includes a UV light screen.

Principal ingredients: Aloe Vera Gel, Caprylic/Capric Triglyceride, Silicone Oil, UV Light Screen, Emulsifier, Emollient Oils, Chamomile Oil.

Drier Skin

As skin ages it tends to become drier, and it loses its youthful bloom, its resilience and elasticity. This is due to decreased sebum production and reduced water-holding capacity.

Recognition

- Dry to the touch
- Early signs of wrinkles around eyes and mouth
- Milia (whiteheads) or closed, blocked pores
- Dilated arterioles — blood vessels that have been stretched through exposure to harsh atmospheres such as heat, sun, wind, cold or central heating without adequate moisturising.
- Dry, flaky patches

This skin type needs products that are oilier and more penetrating than those for younger skin. Vegetable oils have this better penetrating ability and of all natural oils the sweet almond is one of the most beneficial to skin. It is also more resistant to discoloration and rancidity than most vegetable oils. For this reason the Nature's Way range for drier skin utilises sweet almond oil in all the products except the Toner, which uses oils from the blossom.

Salon treatment

1a. Remove all make-up, first with tissue, then you may wish to use Aloe Vera Wash-off Cleansing Gel. Rinse the face, then apply Aloe Vera Wash-off Cleansing Gel on damp cotton wool or with a soft facial brush. Work up a gentle foam, rinse with warm water and gently pat dry.

1b. Alternatively, after removing excess make-up with tissue, you may prefer to use Sweet Almond Cleanser. This rich, creamy product softens the outer horny layers, allowing dry and flaky cells to be gently wiped away with the excess cleanser on tissue.

2. Sweet Almond Enriched Cream Mask should now be applied to further soften and replenish the skin with moisturisers and beneficial oils. Apply a thin layer with a mask brush to the face and neck, leave for 10 to 15 minutes and then remove with cotton wool or tissue.

3. Maintain the skin's natural acid balance by applying pH-buffered, mildly astringent, Sweet Almond Toner.

4. An application of Sweet Almond Moisturiser completes the salon treatment. Massage it gently into the skin until fully absorbed; its rich content of natural oils will maintain the benefits of the first stages of treatment.

5. Eye Gel or Eye Cream with Vitamin E are also recommended as part of the salon treatment. The Eye Gel is slightly astringent with a tightening effect; the Eye Cream is a rich emollient product with Vitamin E.

Treatment summary

1. Cleanse — using Sweet Almond Cleanser or Aloe Vera Wash-off Cleansing Gel.

2. Replenish lost oils and moisture with a 15-minute application of Sweet Almond Enriched Cream Mask.

3. Tone — with gentle Sweet Almond Toner.

4. Moisturise — with Sweet Almond Moisturiser.

5. Foundation — use an oil-based liquid or cream make-up base with added moisturiser.

6. Coverstick — to conceal any dilated arterioles.

7. Use Eye Gel or Eye Cream with Vitamin E.

Home care

Daily:

1. Cleanse, tone and moisturise as for salon treatments, allowing at least 15 minutes before applying foundation over moisturiser.

2. Sweet Almond Night Cream must be applied liberally all over face and neck before going to bed.

3. Extremely dry skins may receive increased benefit from Nature's Way Collagen range.

Weekly:

1. Face mask — Nature's Way Sweet Almond Enriched Cream Mask should be applied liberally to the face and neck area using a clean spatula or mask brush. Relax for 10 to 15 minutes, then remove the mask with damp cotton wool. Tone and moisturise as usual. Do not apply make-up for at least 12 hours.

2. Steam — only to be used if there are very few dilated arterioles; even so, these must be covered. Follow the treatment steps as for oily skin, but essential oil of roses or a handful of rose petals may be added to the water. Steam for 10 minutes to increase circulation, bringing nutrients to the area and speeding away waste products.

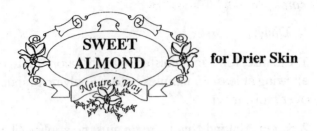

SWEET ALMOND for Drier Skin

Sweet Almond Cleanser

A rich cleansing lotion with almond and other natural oils and beeswax. The pH is adjusted to match the skin's natural acid mantle.

Principal ingredients: Sweet Almond Oil, Beeswax, Magnesium Aluminium Silicate, Sodium Lactate, Caprylic/Capric Triglyceride.

Sweet Almond Enriched Cream Mask

After cleansing, an application of Sweet Almond Enriched Cream Mask protects the skin from vital moisture loss, leaving it soft and supple.

Principal ingredients: Cocoa Butter, Sweet Almond Oil, Polyglycerylmethacrylate, Silicone Oil, Sodium Lactate, Glycerine.

Sweet Almond Toner

A mildly astringent skin toner to close the pores gently and soothe the skin after cleansing. It is pH-adjusted to maintain the skin's natural pH balance.

Principal ingredients: Witch Hazel, Lactic Acid, Ethanol, Glycerine, Almond Blossom Oil, Sodium PCA.

Sweet Almond Moisturiser

User trials have made us acknowledge the attractiveness of cocoa butter in products such as this, and it is included with beeswax, acetylated lanolin alcohol, almond oil, avocado oil and other natural oils chosen for their ability to penetrate the epidermis and promote moisturising of the outer cells. This product is pH-adjusted and the moisturisers are glycerine, sodium PCA and buffered sodium lactate.

Principal ingredients: Almond Oil, Beeswax, Glyceryl Esters, Cocoa Butter, Glycerine, Sodium Lactate, Saturated Emollient Oils, Acetylated Lanolin Alcohol.

NOTE: Lanolin derivatives such as acetylated lanolin alcohol have none of the stickiness sometimes associated with pure lanolin, nor do they have any incidence of allergy reaction or other side effects occasionally attributed to lanolin.

Sweet Almond Night Cream

Seven natural and exotic oils and waxes combined with an advanced humectant system make this a really special product. Throughout the long contact period that a night cream has with the skin's surface, the oils are migrating into the interstitial lipids, softening the epidermis and improving the skin's texture and feel. At the same time, the water-soluble ingredients are being absorbed by the outer cells, thus increasing their moisture-holding capacity.

Principal ingredients: Vitamin E Oil, Wheat Germ Oil, Palm Oil Esters, Grapeseed Oil, Glyceryl Esters, Avocado Oil, Sodium PCA, Caprylic/Capric Triglyceride, Almond Oil, Sodium Lactate, Triethanolamine Stearate.

Dry and Mature or Dehydrated Skin

As the owner ages, skin becomes drier, it loses its elasticity and bounce, the bloom that shines through a youthful skin dulls. Laughter lines become character lines and eventually have to be acknowledged as wrinkles.

This ageing process has many causes: the main reason appears to be that while young skin is abundant in non-cross-linked collagen fibres which are strongly hydrated and elastic, as skin becomes older the degree of cross-linking increases and there is a consequent loss in hydration and elasticity. Lower moisture retention means that the skin is less swollen and the reduced tension results in the skin collapsing into wrinkles. It should be noted that prolonged exposure to sunlight causes severe cross-linking of collagen fibres.

Recognition

- Skin may have crepey appearance.
- Lines and wrinkles apparent.
- Dry, taut feeling, particularly over cheeks and brow bone.
- Loose skin on neck and dropped contours around jaw line.

Salon treatment

1. Cleanse using pure Nature's Way Collagen Cleansing Lotion.

2. Hydrate with Collagen Hydrating Mask, which can be most beneficial to a mature and dehydrated skin after electrical treatments, to hydrate dry and exhausted skin tissue, leaving it soft with improved texture and suppleness.

3. Tone with Nature's Way refreshing Collagen Toner to close pores and maintain the skin's elasticity.

4. Collagen Moisturiser should then be smoothed liberally into the face and neck areas to help to restore the skin's natural vitality.

5. The eye area is frequently very dry and will greatly benefit from an application of Nature's Way Eye Cream with Vitamin E.

6. Necks also become dry with loss of elasticity. Gently massage Nature's Way Neck Cream with Vitamin E and Vegetable Collagen into the neck and throat; use fingertips and a gentle, upward stroking movement.

Home care

Daily:

1. Cleanse with Nature's Way Collagen Cleansing Lotion, massaging gently into face and neck using fingertips. Ensure that any excess is then removed with damp cotton wool.

2. Tone with Collagen Toner, saturating a cotton-wool pad and pressing all over the neck and facial area. Blot dry to prevent soreness.

3. Moisturise, more than once daily if necessary, using creamy Collagen Moisturiser.

4. At night, gently massage rich Collagen Night Cream into the skin with particular attention to dry areas.

5. Apply Eye Cream with Vitamin E to the eye area; carefully avoid the tear duct and do not apply within two hours of going to sleep.

6. Massage Neck Cream with Vitamin E and Vegetable Collagen well into the neck and throat area using fingertips and gentle, upward stokes.

Weekly:

1. Collagen Hydrating Mask should be applied liberally over the face and neck area using a clean spatula. The

mask should be left in position for 10 to 12 minutes before removing excess with tissue and rinsing with tepid water.

2. Tone and moisturise as usual and do not apply make-up for at least 12 hours.

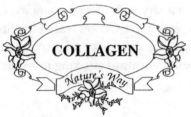

COLLAGEN   **for Dry and Mature Skin**

Collagen constitutes approximately 25 to 30% of the protein content of the human body. It is the support protein of the connective tissue in the shape of fibres which become cross-linked with age. Collagen is the main structural element of the skin and is largely responsible for its characteristic properties.

Biochemically, a collagen fibre is composed of three peptide chains, each with a molecular weight of about 95,000, twisted together to form a super-helix. These triple-helix peptide chains are synthesised in the cutaneous cells or fibroblasts from which they are released into the extracellular spaces where they form aggregates of fibrils, fibres and eventually flat structures.

The use of collagen in skin-treatment products was stimulated by medical investigations into the positive influence of collagen in healing wounds and by investigations into the relationship between age and alterations in the dermal content of collagen.

Unfortunately, because the skin is an effective barrier and collagen molecules are large, it cannot be absorbed through the skin. Its beneficial effects in cosmetics are mainly due to its substantivity to the epidermis and its water-retaining properties. Collagen, as used in cosmetic products, is normally obtained from animal skins, bones and other meat-processing sources. It can be used in either its pure form or as a hydrolysate which renders it water-soluble, although in the latter form its water-retention properties are much reduced.

However, the Nature's Way Collagen range uses vegetable-derived collagen from wheat protein, and whilst it is not a true collagen, it contains the same vital amino acids and exhibits many of the beneficial properties attributed to the animal product. It has good skin substantivity, has excellent moisture-retention properties and preliminary studies show it to increase the firmness of the epidermis and apparently to reduce wrinkling.

The Collagen products are recommended for very dry and mature skin; they are all easy to apply so that delicate tissues are not damaged, and the emphasis is on moisturising and emollience.

Collagen Cleansing Lotion

This is a non-alkaline, skin softening cleanser, enriched with vegetable collagen and sweet almond oil. It has a pH of 5.3 and utilises nonionic emulsifiers to clean the skin thoroughly without drying or irritating it in any way.

Principal ingredients: Collagen, Natural Vegetable Oil, Sweet Almond Oil, Caprylic/Capric Triglyceride, Magnesium Aluminium Silicate, Beeswax, Decyl Oleate.

Collagen Hydrating Mask

A hydrating mask is an excellent way to moisturise and firm the epidermal tissues. This one contains penetrating vegetable oils and cocoa butter for emollience, and lavender oil, renowned for its antiseptic properties, and is fortified with vegetable collagen to moisturise and firm the epidermal tissues.

Principal ingredients: Vegetable Collagen, Cocoa Butter, Lavender Oil, Geranium Oil, Caprylic/Capric Triglyceride, Propylene Glycol.

Collagen Toner

This refreshing lotion with soothing witch hazel and vegetable collagen is used after cleansing and mask treatment to remove residual oiliness and maintain the natural acid mantle.

Principal ingredients: Vegetable Collagen, PEG-6 Caprylic/Capric Triglyceride, Glycerine, Ethanol, Witch Hazel, Sodium Lactate.

Collagen Moisturiser

A well-balanced blend of natural moisturising agents, emollient oils and vegetable collagen for restoring natural vitality to the drier skin.

Principal ingredients: Vegetable Collagen, Beeswax, Acetylated Lanolin Alcohol, Emulsifiers, Natural Oils, Cocoa Butter, Glycerine, Sodium Lactate.

Collagen Night Cream

When mature or dehydrated skin has lost its youthful suppleness and vitality it is essential that a rich night cream be regularly applied to restore gradually its natural elasticity, to prevent further deterioration and to restore earlier good looks. Such a cream is Collagen Night Cream. It contains 5% vegetable collagen in a rich cream base. The oils and waxes have been chosen for their affinity for skin, and they are easy to apply and readily absorbed. A thin film of vegetable collagen and emollient oils is left on the epidermis which, by reducing moisture loss, causes rehydration of the skin.

Principal ingredients: Collagen (Hydrolysed Vegetable Protein), Beeswax, Caprylic/Capric Triglyceride, Sodium PCA, Lavender Oil, Geranium Oil.

Chapter Four

Other Salon-Treatment Products

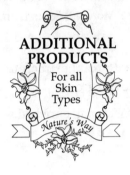

ADDITIONAL PRODUCTS
For all Skin Types
Nature's Way

Eye products

Body products

Ampoules and galvanic therapy

Sun protection

Eye Products

The eyes and surrounding area are particularly vulnerable to mistreatment. The skin on the eyelid is the thinnest part on the whole body. Eyes are prone to bacteriological and fungal infections and the whole eye area is more liable to allergic reactions. For these reasons, special attention must be given to caring for the eyes, and Nature's Way has developed three cleansers and two moisturisers to provide this care.

As with all treatments, until the area to be cared for is clean, a proper assessment cannot be made of the problems and solutions. The eye area is no exception, and Nature's Way has three products to remove eye make-up.

Eye Make-up Remover No. 1 is an oil-based remover for waterproof make-up, applied on dry cotton wool and wiped clean.

Eye Make-up Remover No. 2 is non-oily for sensitive skin; it is applied on damp cotton wool and rinsed off with water.

Eye Make-up Remover Gel in a handy tube; this crystal-clear gel will gently remove all eye make-up including waterproof mascara.

When all traces of eye make-up have been carefully removed, there are two Nature's Way products from which to choose.

Eye Gel is a soothing clear gel with plant extracts to moisturise and tone the delicate eye area.

Eye Cream is a rich and soothing cream, enriched with vitamin E, to hydrate deeply the eye area.

Body Products

Facial Scrub, for all skin types, is a gentle exfoliating scrub to ease away dead hair follicles, emulsified sebum and keratinised cells, leaving the skin glowing with renewed health and vigour.

Body Scrub with a more vigorous action for all-over use, especially on areas of rough skin such as elbows and knees.

Neck Cream with Vitamin E and Vegetable Collagen to hydrate and firm the skin of neck and throat. Highly recommended to accompany the Almond and Collagen ranges.

Hand Cream with cocoa butter, avocado oil and sweet almond oil to care for the hands.

Massage Cream for all-over body massage.

Massage Oil for those who prefer an oil.

Body Contour Cream for areas of fatty tissue and cellulite, especially around the thighs. Plant and seaweed extracts in a penetrating gel of organic silicones to be used daily until treatment is complete. See below for more details on cellulite and its treatment.

Body Conditioning Cream to massage well into all areas that require softening.

Hand and Body Lotion is a light, non-greasy moisturiser for use after bath and shower on the body and all-day application to the hands.

Sun Protect SPF14 is a good UV-A and UV-B protection cream for general protection from the sun and UV light; see p. 65.

Sun Protect SPF 25+, rated "superior" on the Boots Company star rating system for UV-A protection and a total block for UV-B, this is an excellent product for all who are sensitive to sunlight or who wish to protect their skin against harmful UV radiation; see p. 65.

Shower Gel with essential oils for a stimulating shower which will leave the skin soft, smooth and tingle-clean.

Enriched Cream Bath for a long luxurious soak in everlasting, creamy bubbles; with special plant and seaweed extracts, it will leave the skin smooth and soft.

Ampoules for galvanic use and fingertip massage; see p. 62.

Cellulite

"Cellulite! fact or fiction?"; "Cellulite! or is it just fat?". Many magazine articles have appeared under such headings, but there certainly seems to be evidence to support its existence, its effects and its treatment. The root cause of cellulite may be arguable; its appearance in middle age in women that have borne children is common enough.

An excellent article by Kate Hardy in *Les Nouvelles Esthétiques* (Oct./Nov. 1990) describes cellulite as being a degenerative process of the connective tissue. The connective tissue is surrounded by a gel of mucopolysaccharides, protein and water. As cellulite develops this gel-like substance becomes thicker, swelling as it retains water and losing its elasticity. There is a steady accumulation of fluid and toxic waste due to the blood and lymphatic circulatory systems being impaired. Eventually the toxins become trapped under a layer of fibrous tissue creating pockets of water, toxins and fat.

Les Nouvelles Esthétiques also published an article by Dr. Eric-David Aumjaud (Oct./Nov. 1989) which described the medical condition in great detail. He preferred to call the condition "localised lipodystrophy" and he described it in its various forms, some treatable by cosmetics, others of psychosomatic origin or due solely to obesity requiring more specialised treatment.

The visible result of cellulite is the classic "orange peel effect"; other characteristics are a pronounced loss of elasticity and pain caused by the condition.

Various materials are available with which to make anticellulite products, many of which are based on seaweed extracts. Some treatments use electrical currents, galvanism, ionotherapy and faradism; others use a body-wrap technique. All are based on theories of increasing blood flow to the affected area, of breaking up fatty deposits and of removing toxic waste and reducing fluid retention.

The materials which we have examined that appear to be well documented include organic silicones, seaweed extracts and active herbs. Nature's Way has created a product based on these materials, designed to be used with lymphatic drainage techniques and supported by home therapy.

The first treatment must be more in the nature of a consultation. Is the patient obese? What is her age? Has she had children? Does she exercise? Does she smoke or drink alcohol to excess? Success with your treatment will depend very much on the patient's willingness to take your advice and to help herself. When you have identified all the problems and suggested behavioural improvements, it is time to start the treatment with Body Contour Cream. Some therapists prefer to discuss a client's lifestyle while undertaking the massage; the client is usually more relaxed and perhaps more willing to have her problems corrected.

Take a new tube of Body Contour Cream and massage it well into all areas affected by cellulite in order to stimulate lymphatic flow, and explain to the patient your technique. Discuss the need to massage it thoroughly into all affected areas and the actions that she herself can use to continue the therapy at home. Explain that cellulite is globules of fat in the lower dermal layers and how they trap water and toxins in the tissue. Explain how your massage with Body Contour Cream is breaking up these masses, allowing the body's own waste-disposal system to carry them away.

Do not remove the product on completion; it should be completely absorbed and should remain in the dermal tissues to continue its action. Give your client the tube with the remaining product and instruct her to use it daily before retiring, until the contents are exhausted. She should then return to you for inspection, a professional treatment and another supporting course of home treatment. After using one tube there should be a noticeable reduction in pain, increased elasticity and a visible improvement in appearance. However, do not expect miracles and warn your client not to expect them. Cellulite takes years to build up to the stage when treatment is normally sought, and it will not be cured overnight; it will take effort on your client's part for you to be successful.

The series of massage movements shown in the following figure are within the capability of the majority of your clients suffering from cellulite. Massage using the

Body Contour Cream for lubrication will ensure maximum action of the active principals.

1. Using both hands, massage in spiral movements in progressively larger circles to the top of the thighs. This action should continue for 5 minutes per thigh.

2. Using both hands, gently roll folds of flesh from the front of the thighs towards the rear. Repeat the action 5 times on each thigh.

3. Using both hands, place the thumbs together on the inside of the thigh and gently apply pressure at short intervals from the knee to the top of the thigh, repeating this action in turn on both thighs 5 times.

4. Finally, massage in large sweeping circles from the hip down the thigh and back up to the bottom. Continue this action until all the Body Contour Cream is fully absorbed.

A warm bath immediately prior to treatment will increase the blood supply to the affected areas and will be beneficial to the treatment. Using Nature's Way Enriched Cream Bath in the water will make it a very pleasant experience. Each tube should be enough for one professional treatment and six days of home use.

Ampoules and Galvanic Therapy

Galvanic therapy, or electrophoresis, using biologically active materials is an established form of beauty treatment. The process may be used to clean, moisturise, stimulate and regenerate cells.

All treatments commence with a thoroughly cleansed skin, wiped over with a skin toner, to improve current flow; similarly, the electrodes must be thoroughly clean and free of grease.

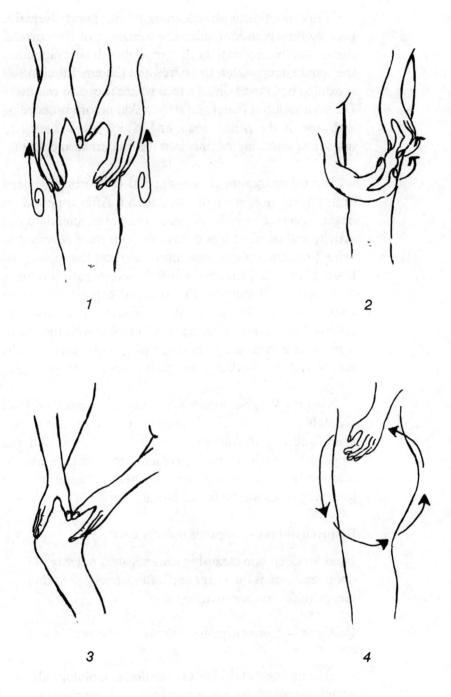

Figure 10. Massage technique

Disincrustation is the cleaning of the pores. Negative polarity only is used. Under the influence of the current, the sodium bicarbonate in the ampoule solution saponifies the sebum deep within the pores and the emulsified result is exuded onto the skin's surface where it can be removed. Disincrustation is beneficial to oily skin before proceeding with any of the other treatments which are designed to introduce active ingredients into the epidermis and dermis.

The other treatments are applied to thoroughly clean skin, possibly following disincrustation. After a period on negative current which will open the pores, stimulate cell activity and increase blood flow, the current is reversed to drive the active ingredients into the receptive epidermal layer. If this dual treatment is followed, reduce the times to a total of 10 minutes. Practice and experience will be your best guide, but start with 5 minutes' disincrustation followed by 3 minutes on negative current with the active ingredient and a final 2 minutes of positive current; this may be reduced further if using aloe vera on sensitive skin.

Nature's Way ampoules are designed to work with all reputable makes of galvanic apparatus and the manufacturer's instructions should be followed. All the ampoules contain active ingredients in a mild, ionisable solution with a slightly alkaline pH. In addition, the following notes will be found useful.

Disincrustation — *negative polarity only*

Used for deep skin cleansing with negative polarity, it opens and cleans the pores and, after rinsing, the skin is receptive for further treatments.

Collagen — *8 mins negative polarity; 2 mins positive polarity*

Used to improve elasticity and to stimulate biological activity. A particularly effective course of treatment is disincrustation followed by Collagen, with the client taking Collagen ampoules home for massaging into the tissues each night, returning to the salon for further treatment after 10 days.

Aloe Vera — *4 mins negative polarity; 1 min positive polarity*

Used for sensitive skins, gently applied and left to continue its healing and moisturising action.

Ginseng — *6 mins negative polarity; 2 mins positive polarity*

Used to stimulate the tissues and refine open pores, leaving the skin glowing with vitality.

Chamomile — *8 mins negative polarity; 2 mins positive polarity*

Used for young, oily skin after disincrustation and of particular benefit in the treatment of acne-damaged skin.

Remember that ampoule products contain highly active ingredients which, when used with care, have spectacular results. It is important to follow the machine manufacturer's instructions and to understand thoroughly the principles involved.

Sun Protection

Until the 1920s it was unfashionable for the white-skinned races to have a suntan, for it was taken to show that the tanned person worked outside on manual tasks. Then the wealthy discovered the pleasures of the French Mediterranean and a suntan became socially acceptable. Sunburn was prevented by wearing light clothing and broad-brimmed hats. Then came the war, and protection was required for men fighting in the deserts and the Pacific. They were issued with red petroleum jelly and zinc oxide pastes — they must have looked rather strange. Efforts were made to find more acceptable protection and, as the understanding of what caused sunburn grew, so did the recognition of chemical sun-screens.

A chemical sun-screen absorbs ultraviolet light. For the next fifty years the requirement was for a material that would absorb the ultraviolet light known to cause sunburn, the so-called UV-B, without blocking the tanning, or UV-A, light. The SPF system was introduced as a guide to how much protection a product would give an individual. It is a factor which is used to multiply the period of a person's natural resistance to give an increased margin of safety. Thus, if a person burns readily and can only go in the sun for 10 minutes before going red, an SPF of 8 would enable him to stay out in the sun for 8 x 10 = 80 mins; if normally a person were safe for an hour, then SPF 8 would give 8 hours protection.

Very few products were sold with a higher value than 8 and, with the continued fashion for sunbathing and a deep tan, users were advised to start their holiday with a high value, i.e. SPF 6 or 8, then to graduate to lower ones, ending with an oil product with minimal protection to give the final fully-cooked look.

However, dermatologists were not so enamoured of sun-worship: they were seeing premature ageing, broken veins and liver spots, and various forms of skin cancer. Professor Ronald Marks of the University of Wales' College of Medicine in Cardiff did much to publicise the problem and he and others also showed that UV-A radiation was not the benign friend it was previously thought to be but actually the worst type of radiation reaching the earth's surface.

Concurrently, concern was expressed about the reactive chemicals used for sun-screens and many were either banned from use in cosmetics or their concentration became strictly limited by statute. In consequence, there was a need for more effective sun-screens that had to be effective over a broader spectrum than hitherto and had to come from a decreased selection of possible ingredients.

Chemists everywhere looked for ways of satisfying this need. One way was for a cocktail of chemicals to provide overlapping ranges of protection, with each material being within the permitted maximum level, and this has proven quite effective, especially for the low-to-medium protection factors.

Another approach was to use microfine titanium dioxide, a very white insoluble pigment, often found in white paint. However, its opacity is related to its particle size, and it has been found that below a certain size titanium dioxide stops transmission of ultraviolet light but allows the passage of visible light: thus there is protection without a noticeable whitening on the skin.

This use of titanium dioxide is a technological breakthrough in skin protection. Formulation with this advanced material is difficult, but after eighteen months of extensive testing, Nature's Way is launching two sun-protection products, Sun Protect SPF 14 and Sun Protect SPF 25+.

Sun Protect SPF 14

Use this smooth, white cream for normal protection from harmful ultraviolet light. It has an SPF of 14 for UV-B light and is rated "good" by the Boots Company star rating system for UV-A radiation. This product is suitable for everyday use by those who wish to protect their skin from harmful ultraviolet light.

Sun Protect SPF 25+

With an SPF of 25+ and rating 3 stars for "superior" protection on the Boots Company star rating system for UV-A light, this product will protect the most delicate complexions from strong sunlight, whether on the beach, the sea or the ski slopes.

Principal ingredients (of both products): Microfine Titanium Dioxide, Caprylic/Capric Triglyceride, Cocoa

Butter, Octyl Palmitate and Propylene Glycol in a water-in-oil emulsion.

If you are on holiday and wish to tan, we suggest using Sun Protect SPF 14 to get acclimatised to the strong sunlight of holiday beaches, then using Nature's Way Aloe Vera Moisturiser which has an SPF of 6 and is an excellent moisturiser.

Chapter Five

Nature's Way Aromatherapy

Aromatherapy is the therapeutic use of aromatic oils obtained from plants. It is inextricably related to perfumery, which uses the same essential oils to create aesthetically pleasing aromas. The story of perfumery is as old as civilisation and some methods of extraction have hardly changed in recorded history. The tomb of Tutankhamen, dated as 1350 B.C., contained alabaster jars of aromatic resins in animal fat. Other Egyptian tombs contained various items related to perfumery and cosmetics, particularly unguent jars and kohl. (There is also a manicure set from the same period.)

On the breast of the Sphinx (1600 B.C.) King Thothmes IV is portrayed offering fragrant oils. The Egyptians used perfumes as offerings to their gods, for personal adornment and for embalming their dead. We can guess the value of their aromatic compounds from the beautiful containers made from such valuable materials as ivory, alabaster and onyx, many of which can be admired in the British Museum.

The ancient Egyptians were the first civilisation to use baths to which they added aromatic oils; bathing was followed by the application of sweet-smelling unguents. Sesame oil, almond and olive oil were the usual vehicles and the aromatic materials included gums and resins and frankincense, myrrh, spikenard, thyme and origanum.

The use of essential oils continued through the ages. The ancient Greeks and Romans used them in bathing, the Crusaders brought back exotic oils and unguents from the Crusades and, as Europeans gravitated towards the cities, the use of aromatic compounds to overcome the noisome odours of populations lacking in personal hygiene became commonplace.

Although the use of essential oils was extensive, it was not until relatively recently that they were used for therapeutic purposes. Elisabeth Jones in *Aromatherapy and Cosmetic Science*[4] dates the modern practice of aromatherapy to the period of the First World War, when Gattefossé, a French chemist, became interested in the medicinal qualities of essential oils and quoted examples of their benefits in the treatment of skin cancer, gangrene osteomalacia and burns. In 1928 he wrote a book called *Aromathérapie*[5] and followed it by many scientific papers relating to therapy by the use of essential oils of plants.

Another Frenchman, Dr Jean Valnet, inspired by Gattefossé's work, used essential oils in the treatment of war wounds during World War II and found them to be exceedingly effective. He too subsequently wrote many books and articles, the best known being the book *The Practice of Aromatherapie*.[6] Since then aromatherapy has gained universal interest and this ancient art, once full of ritual and magic, is now, as we approach the twenty-first century, becoming a modern science.[4]

Natural perfume from plants is due to minute traces of essential oils which can exist in the petals, leaves, stem and roots. These essential oils can be obtained from:

Flowers: cassie, jasmine, mimosa, rose, heliotrope, hyacinth, orange blossom, violet, ylang-ylang, carnation and clove;

Flowers and leaves: lavender, rosemary, peppermint and violet;

Leaves and stems: geranium, patchouli, petitgrain, verbena and cinnamon;

Barks and Woods: cinnamon, cassia, canella, cedar, linaloe and santal;

Roots and rhizomes: angelica, sassafras and vertivert, ginger, oris and calamus;

Fruits: bergamot, lemon, lime and orange;

Seeds: bitter almonds, anise, fennel and nutmeg; and

Gums and resins: from labdanum, myrrh, olibanum, Peru balsam, storax and tolu.

In the same way as wines from different regions and vineyards and of different vintages have distinctive characteristics, so the odours of plants vary with the area of origin, the climate, soil and seasons.

The collection of essential oils is by distillation, expression and extraction. Distillation is one of the oldest methods, the plant material being heated with hot water or steam to release the volatile oil, which is then cooled and collected as a distillate. Expression is a method in which the oils are squeezed from the plant material by force; it is commonly used to obtain citrus oils. Extraction is the removal of essential oils by dissolving them in solvents which are then allowed to evaporate to leave the pure oil. This method is less likely to change the natural material than is distillation.

It can be appreciated why essential oils are so expensive when it is realised that 1000 kg of lavender yield less than 10 kg of oil, 1000 kg of geranium yield less than 1500 g, 1000 kg of rose petals only 500 to 800 g of oil, and that it takes 33 tons of violet petals and leaves to obtain one kilogram of essential oil.

The resins so often referred to in ancient texts are exudates from trees and shrubs, usually as a result of damage to the bark. Myrrh occurs as little tears on the trunks of small trees growing in Saudi Arabia and East Africa. Resins have heavy, often sweet odours; they are used as fixatives to slow down the evaporation of the volatile essential oils.

Because of cost, uncertainties of supply and the impossibility of meeting today's demands from natural sources, many synthetic aromatic substances have been developed for use in perfumery. They can be chemically identical to the principal essential oils found in nature and used to imitate their natural odour or they can be totally different from any naturally occurring material and give a distinctive fantasy smell. A perfume may be entirely synthetic or a blend of natural and synthetic; rarely will it be entirely natural.

The oils used in Nature's Way Aromatherapy products are only from natural sources, for it is only by using the natural essential oil that we can be sure that the full therapeutic value is being obtained. Each oil is a complex mixture and may contain alcohols, phenols, ketones, aldehydes and terpenes. A close study of the chemical composition of the oils reveals why so many are useful in treating wounds and skin complaints. Many are powerful antibiotics; most have a rubefacient effect, stimulating dermal activity; some are local anaesthetics. The molecular size of the ingredients is usually small and they are able both to enter epidermal cells and to pass through the interstitial lipids into the dermis.

In the search for the physical reasons for the success of aromatherapy, Woodruff and Jones (*op. cit.*) realised that the mental reasons were being overlooked. It should be remembered that long before Gattefossé discovered that the phenol content of lavender oil could prevent infection in wounds, lavender was used by herbalists in many of their potions, and posies of the flowers were carried to ward off evil spirits, i.e. what we now know to be the bacteria that causes infection.

Professor Van Toller of the University of Warwick has pioneered work to explain the mental processes in perfume appreciation. Homeopathic medicine uses unbelievably minute traces of active ingredients to treat patients. It is not unrealistic to suppose that the few molecules of an essential oil necessary for an appreciation of its odour can pass through the nasal passages into the lungs and then into the blood stream, and hence affect the brain.

Robert Tisserand (*Essential Oil Safety Data Manual*)[7] warns of the dangers of using essential oils unwisely; in particular they should never be ingested. The oils used are often from culinary herbs, but at a much greater concentration than would be obtained from a few leaves used in food.

The study of essential oils and the art of aromatherapy is fascinating and the value of attending a recognised course in the subject cannot be overstated. Nature's Way has put together a selection of the most useful oils; all are pure, natural oils, carefully checked for quality and bottled correctly in amber glass to improve their keeping. In addition some mixtures have been blended in pure, vegetable carrier oils, readily diluted for use.

Aromatherapy is used in many ways, massage being the most common. The combination of healing hands, odours and oils is a potent one and the sense of relaxed wellbeing after such a treatment is very much part of the therapeutic process. Aromatherapy is not confined to massage, however: the use of essential oils in a face mask or a moisturiser, in the bath or a skin toner, is also highly recommended. Nature's Way has provided some fragrance-free products specially for the addition of essential oils and those who wish to experiment further are urged to read *Aromatherapy and Cosmetic Science*[4] by Woodruff and Jones and other works on the subject (see Bibliography).

The following list is of oils currently available in the Nature's Way range showing the properties each is believed to have when used in aromatherapy. These properties may affect both the mental and physical state; often they have not been confirmed by modern scientific research but have been experienced through centuries of careful use. The principal constituents of each oil are shown and those interested may refer to the list of materials with their proven medical action (see p. 82) in order to relate them to the properties claimed for the essential oil.

Basil *Ocymum basilium*

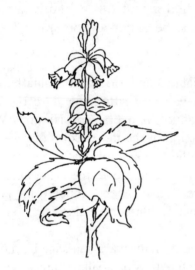

Indigenous to Asia, the oil is distilled from the flowering tops and leaves of the plant. It clears the head, is mentally stimulating and acts as a nerve tonic. It aids clarity of thought and is ideal for revitalising a congested skin or for throat and sinus problems.

Principal constituents: linalol, methyl chavicol, eugenol, limonene and a little citronellol.

NOTE: This oil should be avoided during pregnancy.

Bergamot *Citrus bergamia*

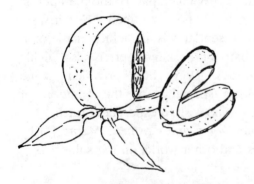

Obtained by expression from the rind of the citrus fruit, this oil has a fresh, spicy, lemon scent. An excellent antiseptic and uplifting nerve tonic, it helps to clear problem skin and aids digestion.

NOTE: Bergamot Oil is phototoxic: do not use it if going into the sun or using a sun-bed and warn clients of the risk.

Parry (*Parry's Cyclopaedia of Perfumery*)[8] gives the principal constituents as linalyl acetate, limonene, pinene, camphene, bornylene and bisabolene.

Chamomile *Matricaria chamomilla*

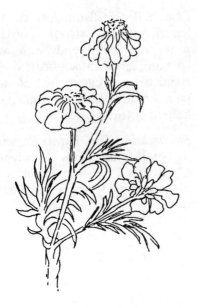

To obtain the oil, chamomile flowers are distilled. The most important ingredient is chamazulene which is reported to soothe sensitive skin and reduce inflammation. It helps penetration of other elements into the skin and has an uplifting effect on depression and anxiety. An important constituent of chamazulene is α-bisabolol which has an antiseptic action. Chamazulene is practically insoluble in water and α-bisabolol has only limited solubility, so the essential oil is more efficacious than the aqueous herbal extract.

Cypress *Cupressus sempervirens*

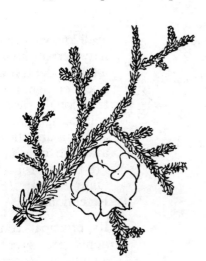

The leaves, flowers and twigs are used. It has a vasoconstrictive effect and is a general astringent; it is also good for refining the pores.

The principal constituent of cypress oil is cedrol, also known as cypress camphor, and it also occurs in cedar wood oil. It is used in perfumery for its spicy-woody note and in aromatherapy for its effects on the respiratory system.

Eucalyptus *Eucalyptus globulus*

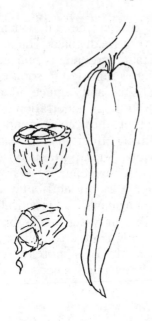

Obtained by distillation of the leaves. It has strong antiviral properties and blends well with lavender as an antiseptic. It is also claimed to relieve aches and pains, reduce fluid retention and help to detoxify the body.

Martindale: The Extra Pharmacopoeia[9] describes eucalyptus oil as 70% cineole; it is very poisonous and used as a rubefacient.

Fennel *Foeniculum vulgare*

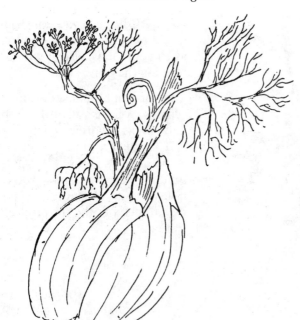

Well known as a culinary herb, it grows as a bushy plant, four to five feet high. It has a traditional use in combating obesity and as a diuretic. It is available only in the Pre-blend for Cellulite and Fluid Retention.

Its principal constituents are given as anethole, fenchone and phellandrene.

Frankincense *Boswellia thurifera*

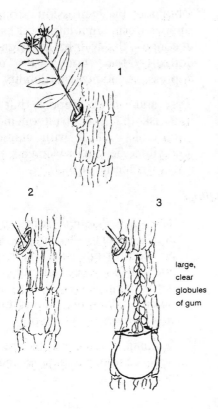

1

2

3

large,
clear
globules
of gum

Available only in the Blend for Stretch Marks, it is exuded from the tree as a gum and has always been highly prized for its scent. It is claimed to lift the spirits and soothe the mind. It is a mild astringent and has regularly found favour in anti-wrinkle preparations, from the Ancient Egyptians to the present day. Parry (*op. cit.*) records how frankincense was exchanged for gold in a barter-ing arrangement by Arabian traders early this century and that the gum was chewed by men who grew tired in the harem!

Parry (*op. cit.*) reports the principal constituents as α-pinene, camphene, dipentene and traces of other alcohols and esters.

Geranium *Pelargonium odorantissimum*

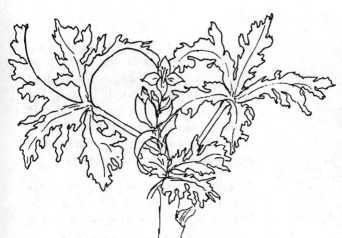

One of the most popular oils. Good for mood swings, it also acts as an anti-coagulant. The fra-grant geranium oil is mainly found in glan-dular hairs on the leaves.

Its principal con-stituents are citron-ellal, geraniol, terpineol, limonene, 5-methoxypsoralen and linalyl acetate.

Grapefruit *Citrus paradisi*

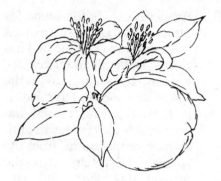

Obtained by expression from the rind. A fresh, stimulating oil used to decongest the lymphatic system and detoxify the body. It uplifts depression and nervous debility.

Tisserand (*op. cit.*) reports that there is a risk that grapefruit oil may be phototoxic; use it with caution if going into the sun or using a sun-bed and warn clients of the risk.

Juniper *Juniperus communis*

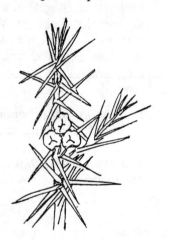

The oil is distilled from the fruit and is used to flavour gin. It can be used for oily skin and is excellent for use on cellulite due to its detoxifying properties and action on circulation and fluid retention. It is a powerful antiseptic.

Its major constituents are borneol, camphene, pinene and terpineol.

Lavender *Lavendula officinalis*

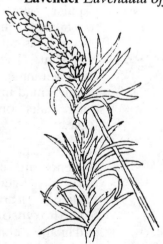

One of the most popular oils, distilled from either the flowers or the whole plant. It promotes healing and cell replacement. It is good for burns, bruises, bites and sunburn. It balances the nervous system and is a mild pain-killer. It is useful for headaches and muscular strains.

Martindale (*op. cit.*) reports that lavender oil contains 35% esters as linalyl acetate and is used as a carminative and insect repellent.

Lemon *Citrus limonum*

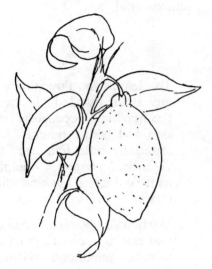

Obtained by expression of the rind, this popular and distinctive oil is an excellent antiseptic. Stimulating and uplifting, it is also good for infections and congested skin.

Its major constituents are citronellal, camphene, limonene and pinene.

NOTE: Lemon oil is phototoxic; do not use it if going into the sun or using a sun-bed and warn clients of the risk.

Lemongrass *Cymbopogon flexuosus* or *Cymbopogon citratus*

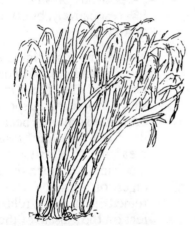

The cultivated variety is known as *Cymbopogon citratus*. It is much used in perfumery for its verbena odour. Its principal constituent is citral (70%) with traces of citronellal, geraniol, linonol and limonene.

Melissa *Melissa officinalis*

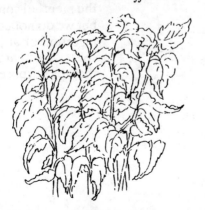

The leaves are distilled, providing a calming, cheering oil. It lowers high blood pressure and is used to treat depression, anxiety or grief.

Nowak[10] gives the major constituents as 40% citronellal, 16% citral, 15% citral b (neral) and 10% caryophyllene, plus linalol, geraniol, sesqiterpenes, triterpenic acids and polyphenols. Its main properties are soothing and antibacterial.

Peppermint *Mentha piperita*

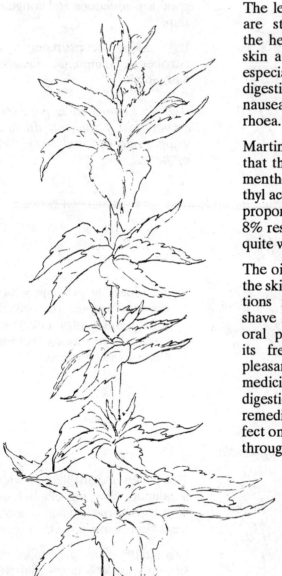

The leaves and flowering tops are steam-distilled. It clears the head and decongests both skin and bodily systems. It is especially effective on the digestive system, helping nausea, indigestion and diarrhoea.

Martindale (*op. cit.*) reports that the main constituents are menthol, menthone and menthyl acetate in the approximate proportions of 45%, 23% and 8% respectively, but these vary quite widely.

The oil has a cooling effect on the skin and is used in preparations for the feet, in aftershave lotions and especially in oral preparations because of its fresh, cooling taste and pleasant after-taste. In medicine it is much used in indigestion and flatulence remedies. It has a relaxing effect on the muscle of the colon through calcium antagonism to the menthol content but we do not advise ingestion of any oils sold for aromatherapy purposes.

Rosemary *Rosmarinus officinalis*

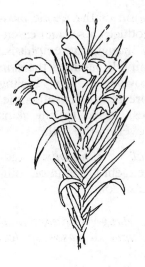

The whole herb is harvested and distilled. It is very stimulating and is thought to improve mental activity. It has a diuretic effect, helping to alleviate fluid retention. It is also valuable for scalp conditions and disorders.

Martindale (*op. cit.*) reports that it contains 2-5% esters as bornyl acetate and 10-18% free alcohols, mostly borneol and linalol, and that its properties are carminative and mildly irritant.

Its stimulating properties are due to its caffeine salts, which also have an antimicrobial action, and its diphenol content, which has an antioxidant action.

Sandalwood *Santalum album*

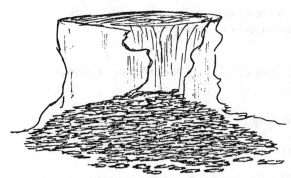

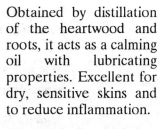

Obtained by distillation of the heartwood and roots, it acts as a calming oil with lubricating properties. Excellent for dry, sensitive skins and to reduce inflammation.

Its principal constituent (95%) is santalol — a sesquiterpene alcohol.

Tea Tree *Melaleuca alternifolia*

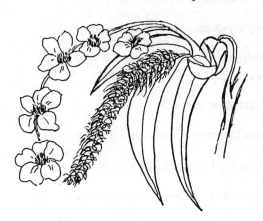

Indigenous to Australia, the oil is obtained by distillation of the leaves. It has antifungal properties and is a good antiseptic, due principally to its high cineole content. Add a few drops to a little Cucumber Toner to cool the feet, dispel odours and for its antifungal action.

Ylang-Ylang *Cananga odorata*

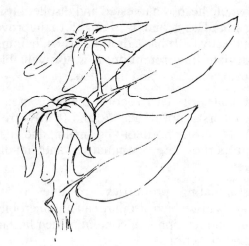

Distillation of the exotic blossom produces a sensual essential oil thought to emphasise femininity. It balances the skin and provides a "safe" feeling for depressed or tense people. It is best suited to oily skins and is lovely in the bath.

Principal constituents: cadinine, eugenol, geraniol, pinene and safrole.

NOTE: Ylang-ylang oil should not be used in cases of dermatitis.

Recognised action of the principal constituents identified in various essential oils.

Anethole Similar to anise oil, carminative and mild expectorant.

Azulene Soothing.

Benzoic acid Antibacterial and antifungal.

Benzyl alcohol Antibacterial and antifungal, local anaesthetic and antipruritic.

Borneol Camphor-related.

Cadinene Antipruritic, keratoplastic, for psoriasis, eczema, seborrhoea.

Camphene Camphor-related.

Camphor Rubefacient and mild analgesic.

Carvacrol Strongly bacteriostatic (thymol isomer).

Caryophyllene Odour midway between cloves and turpentine.

Cineole Very poisonous and a rubefacient. Also known as eucalyptol, it is obtained from cajuput and eucalyptus oil. Used as a counterirritant in ointments and in dentifrices.

Citral Lemon odour but unstable above pH 7.

Citronellal Citrus odour, used as an insect repellent.

Citronellol Odour of rose.

Coumarin Reported to be a macrophage stimulant and has been used with cimetidine in the treatment of melanoma and other tumours.

Cymene Local analgesic applied as an ointment for the relief of rheumatic conditions.

Eugenol Has an odour of cloves, is used as an analgesic in dentistry but can be irritating.

Farnesol Has a sweet floral odour, reminiscent of lilac and cyclamen.

Fenchone Used as a counterirritant, has a warm camphor-like odour.

Geraniol Rose-like odour attracts insects!

Indole Used in perfumery.

Jasmone Jasmine odour.

Limonene Pleasant lemon-like odour.

Linalol or *linalool* Constituent of many essential oils, has bergamot-like odour.

Linalyl acetate Bergamot odour.

Menthol A mild local anaesthetic which is also antiseptic. Used as a topical antipruritic. Incompatible with camphor and phenols. Menthol dilates the blood vessels, giving a cooling sensation and is a local analgesic. It relieves itching and is used as a nasal decongestant but should be used with caution.

Nerol Sweet rose-like odour.

Phenols Germicidal and antibacterial constituent of many oils. Their antibacterial action is reduced in alkaline products and in the presence of cationic surfactants.

Pinene Common constituent of essential oils.

Pulegone Pleasant odour between camphor and peppermint.

Safrole Topical antiseptic with a spicy-floral odour present in many essential oils.

Santalol. Sesquiterpene alcohol and major constituent (95%) of sandalwood oil.

Sesqiterpenes and *Terpenes* Many of the essential oils contain unsaturated alcohols, that is, they have a double bond and a -CH_2OH group. These are known as terpenes and are largely responsible for the characteristic odour of the plant from which the oil has been extracted. Such terpenes are citronellol, geraniol, nerol, linalol and farnesol, which is a sesquiterpene.

Terpineol Used as a disinfectant.

Thymol This is 2-isopropyl-5-methyl-1-phenol or isopropyl metacresol. Strong antimicrobial but irritant and largely inactivated by protein.

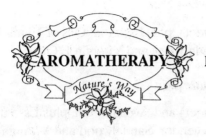 **Facial and Body Massage Oils**

Three ready-blended facial massage and five body massage oils are available. Each massage oil is a delicate blend of essential oils in a carrier oil with added vitamin E which helps prolong the life of the blend.

For Arthritis and Rheumatism

Almond Oil (Sweet), plus Essential Oils of Eucalyptus, Juniper, Rosemary and Vitamin E.

For Body Aches and Pains

Grape Seed Oil plus Essential Oils of Juniper, Lavender, Bergamot and Vitamin E Oil.

For Relaxing Bodily Stress

Grape Seed Oil plus Essential Oils of Chamomile, Juniper, Melissa and Vitamin E Oil.

For Cellulite and Fluid Retention

Grape Seed Oil plus Essential Oils of Juniper, Rosemary, Fennel and Vitamin E Oil.

For Stretch Marks

Avocado Oil plus Essential Oils of Frankincense, Lavender, Lemongrass and Vitamin E Oil.

For Oily and Problem Skin

Grape Seed Oil plus Essential Oils of Lemon, Bergamot, Lavender and Vitamin E Oil.

For Dry and Sensitive Skin

Almond Oil (Sweet), plus Essential Oils of Ylang-Ylang, Chamomile, Sandalwood and Vitamin E Oil.

For Dry and Mature Skin

Almond Oil (Sweet) and Avocado Oil, plus Essential Oils of Geranium, Lavender, Sandalwood and Vitamin E Oil.

Carrier Oils

The carrier oil used to dilute the essential oils is an important part of aromatherapy. The use of mineral oils is not suitable. Nature's Way has selected four natural oils, stabilised them with natural vitamin E against rancidity and offers them in useful 250 ml and 500 ml sizes. To use for massage, take sufficient carrier oil and add to it the essential oils of your choice to achieve the desired effect. For a more complete description of these oils, refer to chapter 8.

Avocado Oil Obtained from the flesh of the avocado pear, *Persea gratissima*. It has a very rich skin-feel and will prolong the massage time.

Grape Seed Oil Obtained from the seeds of muscat raisins, this is a lighter oil than the others and may be mixed with them to achieve exactly the consistency sought.

Sweet Almond Oil The fixed oil obtained from *Prunus communis*, also known as *Amygdalus communis*. This oil has always been used in cosmetics because of its pleasant skin-feel and resistance to rancidity.

Wheat Germ Oil Obtained by expression from wheat germ, it is a yellow-to-amber coloured oil with a characteristic odour. It has a rich, oily feel on the skin. Not all aromatherapy treatments use oils for massage. Nature's Way has created two additional products — a Facial Massage Cream and a Face Mask Base.

Facial Massage Cream

A lovely, soft massage cream specially created for facial massage. Use a spatula to remove sufficient for a full facial massage. Place the cream into a suitable container and add a few drops of your selected essential oils to it, mix gently and use for treatment.

Principal ingredients: Almond Oil and Cocoa Butter in a smooth emulsion.

Aromatherapy Mask Base

A soft gel mask makes an excellent vehicle for bringing essential oils into prolonged contact with the skin. Choose your oils with care from the Nature's Way selection chart and add a few drops to the Mask Base as described for the Facial Massage Cream.

Apply the Mask for 10 to 15 minutes, remove excess with tissue and leave the residue to continue caring for the skin. Remember that essential oils are powerful stimulants and that all Nature's Way oils are totally pure, so use sparingly.

Principal ingredients: Glycerine, Aloe Vera and Witch Hazel in a soft, moisturising gel.

Aromatherapy and Essential Oils User Guide

		Stimulates and uplifts
HEAD	Ear/headache	Basil Eucalyptus Lemon
	Toothache	
	Migraine	Basil
	Throat	Bergamot Lemon Tea Tree
	Catarrh	Basil Bergamot Lemon
	Flu	Bergamot Eucalyptus Lemon
	Sinus	Bergamot Eucalyptus Lemon
	Colds	Basil Bergamot Tea Tree
	Asthma	Basil Lemon
	Dandruff/scalp	
SKIN	Hypersensitive	
	Dry	
	Oily	Bergamot Lemon
	Congested	Basil Lemon
	Acne	Bergamot
	Irritated	
	Bites/stings	Basil Bergamot Tea Tree
	Burns	
	Sunburn	
	Dermatitis/eczema	Bergamot
	Psoriasis	Bergamot
	Herpes	Lemon

Affects body systems	*Relaxes and soothes*
Chamomile Lavender Melissa Peppermint	
Chamomile	
Chamomile Lavender Melissa Peppermint	
Cypress Geranium	Sandalwood
Peppermint	Sandalwood
Cypress Chamomile Lavender Peppermint	Sandalwood
Lavender Peppermint	
Peppermint	
Lavender Melissa Peppermint Rosemary	
Juniper Rosemary	
Chamomile	Sandalwood
Chamomile Geranium Lavender	Sandalwood Ylang–Ylang
Cypress Geranium Juniper	Ylang–Ylang
Geranium Peppermint Rosemary	
Chamomile Juniper Lavender	
Peppermint	Sandalwood
Lavender Melissa Peppermint	
Chamomile Geranium Juniper Lavender	
Lavender	
Chamomile Geranium Juniper Lavender	
Lavender	

Stimulates and uplifts

BODY FUNCTIONS	High Blood Pressure	Lemon
	Circulation	Lemon
	Lymphatic congestion	Grapefruit
	Fluid retention	Eucalyptus
	Gastro–enteritis	Basil Bergamot Tea Tree
	Indigestion	Basil Bergamot Tea Tree
	Digestion	Bergamot Eucalyptus
	Cystitis	Bergamot Eucalyptus
	Urinary	Bergamot
	Kidneys	Lemon
	Thrush	Tea Tree
	Diarrhoea	Eucalyptus
	Nausea	
	P.M.T	
	Aches and pains	Bergamot Eucalyptus
	Rheumatics	Eucalyptus Lemon
	Cramp	Basil
	Cellulite	
NERVOUS	Anxiety	Basil Bergamot
	Irritability	
	Nervous debility	Basil Grapefruit
	Depression	Basil Bergamot Grapefruit
	Tension	Basil Bergamot
	Insomnia	Basil

Affects body systems	Relaxes and soothes
Melissa	Ylang–Ylang
Cypress Geranium Juniper	
Cypress Lavender Rosemary	
Geranium Juniper Rosemary	
Chamomile Lavender Peppermint	Ylang–Ylang
Chamomile Juniper Lavender Melissa	
Chamomile Rosemary	
Juniper Lavender	Sandalwood
Geranium Juniper	Sandalwood
	Sandalwood
Chamomile Cypress Peppermint Rosemary	Sandalwood
Lavender Melissa Peppermint	Sandalwood
Chamomile Geranium Lavender Melissa	
Chamomile Juniper Lavender Melissa	
Chamomile Juniper Lavender Rosemary	
Chamomile Cypress Geranium	
Juniper Lavender Rosemary	Sandalwood
Chamomile Juniper Lavender Melissa	
Chamomile Lavender	Sandalwood
	Sandalwood Ylang–Ylang
Chamomile Geranium Lavender	Sandalwood Ylang–Ylang
Juniper Lavender Melissa	Sandalwood Ylang–Ylang
Chamomile Juniper Lavender	

Courses in aromatherapy

All interested in the practice of aromatherapy are strongly advised to attend a recognised course on the subject. A glance through the advertisements in *Health & Beauty Salon* magazine will reveal many excellent courses. Of particular note are the two-day introductory workshops by Elisabeth Jones and John Woodruff on Aromatherapy and Cosmetic Science. In addition, Bellitas Ltd. organise short courses in locations throughout the country, including beauty colleges by arrangement, and can advise on full-length courses leading to recognised qualifications.

For further details contact Bellitas Ltd. (at the address given at the front of this book) or Elisabeth Jones, c/o the Secretary, The Elisabeth Jones College, Blakes House, Upton, Nr Hurstbourne Tarrant, Andover, Hants. Telephone 0264-76384.

A list of books which are essential reading for those interested in aromatherapy is given in the Bibliograpy.

Chapter Six

The Creation of a Skin-Care Product

Every ingredient in a Nature's Way product is there to fulfil the product's purpose. This is not always true of other brands, and many preparations on the market have ingredients included in minute amounts for the sake of a spurious label claim.

Each skin-care product is created for a special effect and this is achieved by a combination of ingredients. Thus in an emulsion there may be several different oils, each labelled "emollient" in one-line descriptions, but all included for their combined properties: one may dry quickly, another penetrate the epidermis, the third may be present to make the product more viscous and easier to apply.

Some materials are present in the product because they are beneficial to the user, others make the product more pleasant to use, while a third group is essential to the keeping properties of the product, e.g. preservatives and magnesium sulphate.

It must be stressed that many ingredients cannot be considered in isolation: sometimes they combine chemically with other constituents, sometimes their effect in one product is quite different from that in another. Triethanolamine is a commonly listed material, but it is rarely present as such in the product since it is frequently used to neutralise an acid such as stearic acid or a carbomer to form a gel.

It may be noticed that one product has one or two preservatives, and that another product has a quite different preservative system. This is usually because so many preservatives are inactivated in certain systems. Methylparaben, for example, is inactivated by polysorbate 20. When a triethanolamine stearate emulsion turns out too thick, it can often be thinned by the addition of polysorbate 20, but this may render the preservative system ineffective.

To illustrate the way in which materials are used to develop a formulation, the following is a description of how Nature's Way Neck Cream with Vitamin E and Vegetable Collagen was created. The need for a neck cream was identified, as one was not available in the Nature's Way range. In consultation with salon owners and advisers, the type of product required, the skin type for which it was intended and the way in which it would complement the existing ranges of products were discussed in detail.

It was decided that a rich massage-type cream was required that could be gently massaged into the neck. It would frequently be applied at night and left *in situ* until morning to keep the active ingredients in close contact with the skin for a long period. It could be considered too greasy for normal daytime use unless the user had particularly dry skin. Such a product would have a high oil content and would be best applied as a water-in-oil emulsion.

A high oil content allows an occlusive film to form on the skin, preventing skin perspiration and improving moisture retention by preventing the skin from losing its natural water content. By making the cream oily, it would require massaging to ensure that it was fully absorbed, and this massage action would be part of the therapy. However, dry skin has lost much of its resilience and elasticity, so the product needed to be very readily applied with the fingers and not drag in any way.

A water-in-oil emulsifier known as pentaerythritol was selected to be used in combination with cetearyl alcohol, which is a greasy, wax-like material. The emulsion formed is not very stable, so PEG-45/dodecyl glycol copolymer was included as a secondary emulsifier. Mineral oil provided the occlusive film and isostearyl alcohol added some skin-penetrating properties. Now the product was too greasy, so the mineral oil was exchanged for caprylic/capric triglyceride, which is a good emollient without the greasiness of mineral oil. However, now the product had become too soft, so beeswax was introduced to give it body.

The product was to contain vitamin E, so this was included; it is an effective material for improving the quality of skin for it has moisturising and free-radical scavenging properties. There are several oils in the product that could suffer from oxidation, so a little antioxidant (BHA) was added; then we remembered that this should not be necessary because of the natural antioxidant effect of the vitamin E, so we removed it.

Having put together the oil phase, we then looked at the aqueous phase. First it needed water, then some humectant to prevent the product from drying out: we included propylene glycol because it is also a skin moisturiser. Sodium lactate was included because of its proven moisturising properties. The skin releases its own sodium lactate as part of the skin's pH-buffering and natural moisturising factor; we were just providing a little more. After initial testing, sodium PCA was added as an additional boost to the moisturising action. It was also decided to include vegetable collagen to further improve the moisturising and skin-feel properties.

Magnesium sulphate was included to improve the stability of the product, and finally were added a fungicide and a preservative to prevent microbiological spoilage and essential oils of lavender, geranium and ylang-ylang for their therapeutic benefits and pleasant aroma.

The product was tested in salons and colleges and refinements made to the proportions of constituents until eventually all were satisfied. At the same time laboratory batches were made and stability-tested under extreme conditions of heat, cold and sunlight until we could be sure of the long-term stability of the product.

Chapter Seven

Hints and Tips for Selling in the Salon

Many therapists have a successful practice but sell very few products to their clients. Others make substantial profits from the products they sell. Why the difference?

The most common reason given by the first group is that the therapist's professionalism is compromised by selling products from the salon.

The second most commonly advanced objection to selling is the fear that if clients can treat themselves at home they will not spend money with the therapist.

To answer the first objection, it is our carefully considered opinion that the therapist is using her professional skills when she advises the client what products to use just as much as when she is treating the client herself. All clients will use a number of products, some good, some quite unsuitable. All Nature's Way ranges have been carefully designed to be a complete treatment with a well-balanced, comprehensive selection of products. It is far better that the client uses products that are correct for her and complementary to the treatment that she is receiving from you than that she uses a preparation that could undo the good that you are achieving.

With regard to the concern about losing a client, many of the treatments need a careful daily routine with a more intensive treatment weekly. Clients do not have the time or money to come to the salon daily; it is far better that they follow your instructions between visits and come to you for the more intensive treatment and a progress check. If your treatment is seen to be successful your client will always come to your salon.

Many people find it hard to sell. They do not like being "pushy"; they are concerned about the client's financial state; they feel that if the client has to pay for products as well as the treatment, the client may consider the total cost of the treatment too much for a repeat visit.

These sentiments are understandable. However, during the course of a treatment the client will usually inquire what products are being used. Often a client will not realise that the same products can be made available to her for home use. Remember that Nature's Way products are sold only through salons, so the client may well never have seen a Nature's Way product before.

Almost all clients will already be buying products for home use. You can sell her Nature's Way products in the full confidence that the products are of excellent quality and good value for money. Keep a record of what products your client purchases at each visit; when you think a product is nearly used up, politely ask whether this is so; it will surprise the client that you can remember what she purchased and estimate how much has been used.

Because greasy skin is usually associated with oily hair, dry skin with dry hair, etc., there is a complementary range of hair products for home use. For each skin type a shampoo and a conditioner are recommended. These hair products are made to the same high standards as the skin-care products and can be recommended and used with confidence.

In order to help you make sales and improve your profits, and as a support to your salon treatment, Nature's Way has devised the following ten-point sales plan.

Nature's Way Ten-Point Sales Plan

1. Prepare your salon and yourself

- Display Nature's Way products in areas that are easily seen — near to your working area or on or near the reception desk.
- Keep the products clean, tidy and clearly priced.
- Learn all you can about the products you are going to sell.
- Create a selling environment in the salon.
- Have the stock!
- Know your client's name and keep a record of her skin type.

2. Present the features of the products

- Nature's Way products are natural products.
- All Nature's Way products are produced and tested without cruelty to animals.
- Nature's Way products are used professionally by you in the salon.
- Attractively packaged, good quality and value for money.
- Mention the products' contents, e.g. almond oil, cocoa butter, vegetable collagen, pure lemon juice, witch hazel, aloe vera gel.

3. Tell them the product's benefits

- Nature's Way will keep them looking younger.
- Nature's Way for healthy skin.
- Helps to restore essential moisture to the skin.
- pH-balanced.
- Natural materials.
- Replenishing, soothing, improves the skin's texture, etc.

4. Presentation

- Select a range of Nature's Way products which suit the customer's skin.
- Place them before her and encourage her to pick them up and ask you questions about them.

5. Look out for buying signals

- Can I buy it here?
- Do you have all the Nature's Way range in stock?
- Do you sell Nature's Way range for home use?
- How much are they?
- Which Nature's Way product is suitable for my skin?
- Can I pay by cheque?
- Do you think it will work on my skin?
- I usually use.....
- Do you find it successful?
- My friend has tried it and said it was nice.

6. Close the sale

- Would you like to take some now?
- Will you try some/one/it?
- Which do you prefer?
- If you take three Nature's Way products for your skin and the Enriched Foam Bath, these will come to .....
- Which product do you think is best for you?

7. Objections

- Listen to them sympathetically, don't take criticism personally. Give a good impression, be friendly and calm.
- Offer a solution.

8. Major objections

- It's rather expensive.
- It's too cheap to do any good.
- It's cheaper at the chemists.
- It's not for me.
- I don't buy products in salons.
- I'm going to grow old gracefully.
- I've always had..........
- Perhaps next time.
- I can't afford it.

9. Learn to spot common objections and practice answers to them

10. Know when to stop

Chapter Eight

Glossary of terms and descriptions of all ingredients used in Nature's Way products

The following glossary is a complete list of ingredients that are currently used in Nature's Way products. Important ingredients are described in depth; others, such as preservatives, pigments and emulsifiers, are described under a common heading. In addition, many of the terms such as *pH, acid mantle* and *natural moisturising factor* used in the text are explained more fully.

In chapter 2, The Cosmetic Care of Skin, Nature's Way products are briefly described and their principal ingredients shown. The materials listed are those that are of particular benefit or thought to be of special interest to the therapist or user. Chapter 9 contains a complete list of all ingredients in each product. The majority of names shown are those currently approved by the Cosmetic, Toiletry and Fragrance Association (CTFA) for listing on products distributed in America, where ingredient labelling is mandatory, although occasionally we have used names more commonly employed in Europe. Eventually the European Community is to introduce compulsory ingredient labelling and some names may change.

In this chapter all materials used in Nature's Way products are described with information on their origin, application and usefulness. The information has of necessity to be brief but it should help the reader to acquire a better understanding of cosmetic chemistry and how it relates to the products that are used in skin care.

Caution is needed in interpreting CTFA and generic names in formulations because these names do not necessarily specifiy a unique material. For example, various glyceryl stearates are available — one form may be used as an emulsifier in low pH systems, another in products of pH 7.0 and above, and yet a third to stabilise a water-in-oil emulsion — all having the same CTFA name but known to the formulating chemist by their diverse trade names.

Glossary

Acetylated Lanolin Alcohol. If lanolin alcohol is treated with acetic anhydride, acetylated lanolin alcohol is obtained. This material is insoluble in water but is alcohol- and oil-soluble. It is particularly useful in reducing stickiness and drag in oily products, and in improving spreadability and penetration of the stratum corneum.

Acid Mantle. Skin is naturally acidic and this acidity is called the acid mantle. The skin of new-born babies has a neutral pH, but it gradually changes during the first week until it reaches a value between 4.5 and 6. The cause of this acidity is the presence of organic carboxylic acids, mainly lactic, pyrrolidine carboxylic and urocanic acids, which form salts with sodium, potassium and ammonium ions. The presence of a weak acid with its salt creates a buffer (q.v.) which maintains an equilibrium pH, resistant to change.

The acids are part of the sebum exudate; the salts are present in perspiration. Not all skins have an identical pH nor do all parts of the body have the same pH. A dry skin is deficient in sebum and may have a higher pH; areas where sweat is prevented from evaporating also have a higher pH; the eye area is near to neutral. A pH value between 5.3 and 5.5 is accepted as the average for normal, healthy skin.

The usefulness of this acid mantle is still being argued. What is accepted is that lactic acid, sodium lactate, pyrrolidine carboxylic acid and sodium pyrrolidine carboxylate are essential constituents of the skin's natural moisturising factor or NMF (q.v.).

Almond Oil. Known as sweet almond oil to differentiate it from the essential oil of bitter almonds. It is the fixed oil obtained from *Prunus communis*, also known as *Amygdalus communis*. The almond belongs to the same group of plants as the rose, plum and peach. The tree is a native of Asia and North Africa but is now cultivated all over the world. It is about 25 feet in height, with pointed, serrate leaves and has a profusion of pink flowers; the oil is obtained from the nut kernel.

Almond oil has always been a common constituent of cosmetics because of its excellent keeping properties. In cheaper products it has been replaced with mineral oil but is much used in Nature's Way products because of its skin softening and soothing properties and its resistance to rancidity. Its principal constituents are the glycerides of oleic and linoleic acids plus a little palmitic acid and myristic acid.

Aloe Vera Gel. The aloe used for cosmetic application is *Aloe barbadensis*, also known as aloe vera, or true aloe. It grows in both tropical and desert areas, but the aloe used in cosmetics is mostly cultivated in the desert regions of Arizona, the Rio Grande area of southern Texas and Florida, Mexico and Guatemala.

The plant is a member of the lily family and closely related to the yucca. It is well known for its laxative effects. Research is currently under way to examine other possible medicinal uses, and some success has been claimed for its antiviral properties. Work at the Southwest Institute for Natural Sources at Grande Prairie, Texas, shows that the gel removed from inside the leaves promotes human cell growth, whereas the sap taken from the outer green leaf-rind is cytotoxic. The growth-promoting factor is due to its concentration of lectins, which are haemagglutinating proteins from the mucopolysaccharides present in aloe vera gel.

In cosmetics we always refer to aloe vera gel, although the gel-like mass found in the freshly harvested leaves is actually a liquid held in a fibrous matrix. The fibre is not cosmetically useful, so the juice is removed by pressing. It then undergoes high-pressure membrane filtration to remove bacteria and purification to remove anthraquinones. The resulting liquid is colourless to pale amber and has a natural pH of between 4.0 and 5.0. It is still termed a gel although water-thin. It has a total solids content of 0.50%, much of which are mucopolysaccharides — large molecules with the ability to retain moisture. There appears to be some proof that the enzyme content of the gel can promote healing.

Amphoteric. See under Surfactants.

Anionic. See under Surfactants.

Antipruritic. From the Latin *pruritis*, "itching"; an antipruritic material alleviates this urge. The desire to scratch can be a response to contact dermatitis, to parasites, to drugs, both illegal and legal, and to chronic disorders ranging from carcinoma to blood disorders. Thus if a client complains of a persistent itch, medical advice should be sought. If it is not due to a serious medical problem, it may be alleviated by the use of an emollient cream: Aloe Vera Night Cream and the Eye Cream with Vitamin E are particularly recommended.

Arterioles. Arteries lead to arterioles which branch into capillaries. Dilated arterioles are blood vessels which have been stretched through exposure to harsh atmospheres such as heat, sun, wind, cold or central heating without adequate moisturising — the familiar red veins of middle age.

Avocado Pear Oil. Obtained from the flesh of the avocado pear, *Persea gratissima*, of which as much as 30% may be extractable oil. The fruit is first dehydrated in an inert atmosphere at 130°C followed by pressing. Although expensive, approximately ten times the cost of mineral oil, it is used in Nature's Way products for its excellent skin-feel properties. It contains vitamins A and B and lecithin; the bulk of the oil consists of glycerides of oleic acid (77%) and linoleic acid (11%).

Azulene. Azulene gets its name from its intense blue colour. It is a constituent of fresh chamomile oil and historically has anti-inflammatory and soothing properties.

Beeswax. Beeswax must take first place in any list of cosmetic waxes. Used by Galen in his famous cold cream, it has been used in cosmetics ever since. It is obtained from the honeycomb and consists of a hard waxy secretion. It is a complex mixture of hydrocarbons, fatty acids and fatty acid esters. Naturally it is yellow, but bleached varieties are more frequently used and are of less strong odour.

Beeswax is regularly used in lipsticks and other solid products and as an emulsifier when combined with borax in cosmetic creams. Cold creams may contain 15 to 20% beeswax but it is more commonly used at 1 to 5% as a viscosity modifier and emulsion stabiliser. Creams with a high beeswax content are notoriously difficult to perfume, rose being one of the few fragrances that blend with its natural odour.

BHA. Butylated hydroxyanisole, or BHA, is an antioxidant. Natural oils undergo oxidation and may become rancid. An antioxidant preferentially absorbs dissolved oxygen, thereby retarding this process. Vitamin E is a natural antioxidant and used wherever possible in Nature's Way products.

Buffers. Normally, if an acid is added to water the pH of the solution varies greatly with concentration. However, if a salt of that acid is also present, large changes in the acid concentration only cause small changes in pH. Buffer action is most effective when applied to a weak acid and its salt, and it is such acids that interest us in cosmetic science.

With both acid and salt in solution the salt completely dissociates and the concentration of the common ion inhibits dissociation by the acid. Thus the acid effect is suppressed and large changes in acid concentration will only cause minor changes in pH. However, the acid is still there in solution and if required to take part in a chemical reaction it is available.

A buffer can be considered as a reserve acid supply. Alkaline buffers are also used and act as a reserve supply of alkali. Examples of the usefulness of this concept are boric acid with sodium borate (borax), which is used to buffer eye-wash lotion at pH 7.3, and lactic acid in conjunction with sodium lactate to adjust the pH of skin toners to between 5.0 and 5.5.

The skin has a natural buffering action which will resist changes due to low levels of topically applied material at a different pH. It is estimated that the skin will always attain its original pH within three hours of application of material of widely differing pH.

Camphor Oil. Only the white camphor oil should be used in cosmetics. It is obtained by steam distillation of *Cinnamomum camphora* trees. It is a rubefacient and has antiseptic and antipruritic properties and acts as a direct cutaneous stimulant[11]. When applied to the skin there is a feeling of warmth and a slight anaesthetic action. It is frequently used in products for the relief of rheumatism. In Nature's Way products it is used for its cutaneous-stimulating properties.

Caprylic/Capric Triglyceride. This oily component is of natural origin, it being derived from coconut and palm kernel oil. Unfortunately, although cosmetically beneficial, the natural oils are prone to rancidity, malodours and discoloration. To keep the benefits without the disadvantages natural oils are distilled to purify them and the distillate is then esterified with glycerine which prevents oxidation and rancidity. Being very pure, this oil is unlikely to cause allergic reactions, whereas a few people are allergic to the oxidation products of natural oils.

Carbomer. A synthetic thickening agent, it is an acidic carboxyvinyl polymer which, when dissolved in water and neutralised with an alkali, such as triethanolamine, forms a clear gel. In Nature's Way products it is frequently used as an emulsion stabiliser as it is little affected by heat. In low concentration it has a pleasant skin-feel and by holding moisture to the skin in a thin film it has some moisturising properties.

Cationic. See under Surfactants.

Cellulite. A disorder of the the subcutaneous connective tissue, characterised by localised excess of fatty deposits and an accumulation of toxins and body fluids associated with poor circulation. (See p. 59 for more details of its cause and treatment.)

Cetearyl Alcohol. Not a drink but a waxy solid obtained from palm oil. Originally it was obtained from tallow, but only cetearyl alcohol of vegetable origin is used in Nature's Way products. It is a common constituent of emulsions, giving them body and a rich feel but too much can be greasy except in hydrating masks and massage products where the greasiness is an advantage. It is a secondary emulsifier and helps to soften creams and improve their application.

Cetearyl Octanoate. An ester (q.v.) obtained by reacting cetearyl alcohol with octanoic acid.

Cocoa Butter. A brittle, wax-like solid at room temperature, it melts at a little below body heat, making it an excellent wax for giving body and texture to a cream which will readily apply to the skin. It consists mainly of the triglycerides of palmitic, stearic and oleic acids with small quantities of arachidic and linoleic acids. It is obtained from the roasted seeds of *Theobroma cacoa*.

Cocoamphocarboxyglycinate. A well proven, very mild surfactant, developed specifically for use in baby products and for products that may come into contact with the eye.

Collagen — animal. Biochemically, a collagen fibre is composed of three peptide chains, each with a molecular weight of about 95,000, twisted together to form a super-helix. These triple-helix peptide chains are synthesised in the cutaneous cells or fibroblasts, from which they are released into the extracellular spaces where they form aggregates of fibrils, fibres and eventually flat structures.

Collagen — vegetable. Collagen is described in detail in the introduction to the Collagen range for Dry and Mature Skin.

DEA-Oleth-3 Phosphate. An emulsifier (q.v.). Stable at acid pH and exceptionally skin-friendly.

Decyl Oleate. An ester (q.v.).

Denatonium Benzoate. Also known by its trade name "Bitrex", it is claimed to be the most bitter substance known to man. Denaturants, such as denatonium benzoate, are mandatory ingredients in any cosmetic-grade ethanol, to prevent human consumption.

Dimethicone. Also known as silicone oil, this inert material is deposited on the skin from a cosmetic emulsion to give it a soft, smooth feel without stickiness. It provides excellent water repellency and protection against water and airborne irritants.

Disodium EDTA. Some synthetics are unavoidable. Disodium EDTA is a chelating agent, suppressing the effects of iron contamination in skin toners and increasing preservative efficacy in some other products.

Elastin. Like collagen, elastin is an essential component of the connective tissue and is largely responsible for its elasticity. The two materials always occur in nature interlaced, the proportions dependent on the nature of the organ, those that stretch and contract frequently having the highest level of elastin. The aorta is 30 to 45% elastin, the lungs 10 to 15%, ligaments in the neck of a bull are about 80% elastin but skin has only about 5% elastin content.

Although the elastin content of the skin is relatively low it is extremely important, allowing the skin to move freely with the limbs and yet retaining it as an elastic covering. The interlacing of collagen fibres with elastin fibres in a lubricating bed of mucopolysaccharide gel gives the skin its suppleness, elasticity, tenacity and strength and its softness and smoothness.

Emulsions and **Emulsifiers.** All Nature's Way cleansing lotions, moisturisers and night creams are emulsions. An emulsion is a stable mixture of oils and water, either minute droplets of oil surrounded by the water phase — an oil-in-water emulsion — or minute droplets of water surrounded by the oil phase — a water-in-oil emulsion.

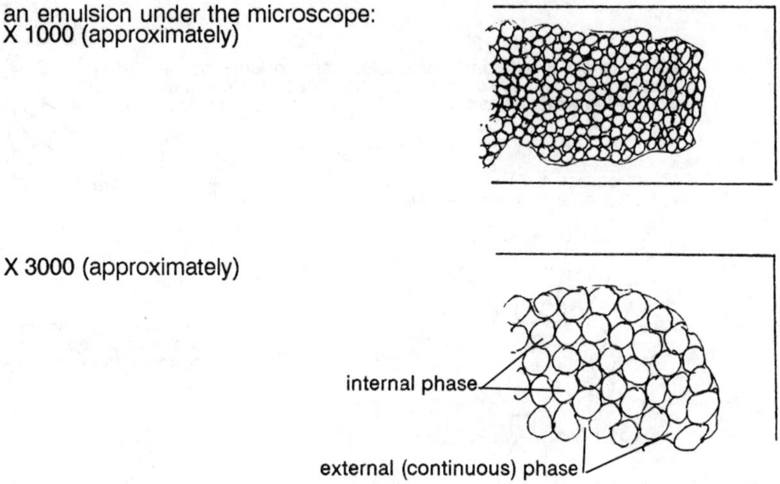

an emulsion under the microscope:
X 1000 (approximately)

X 3000 (approximately)

internal phase

external (continuous) phase

Figure 11. Structure of an emulsion (diagrammatic)

In either case, the oil phase contains all the oils and waxes and oil-soluble components. The aqueous phase contains all those items that are water-soluble such as herbal extracts, moisturising agents, gums and thickeners.

An emulsion is a much improved vehicle for applying active ingredients to the skin than by simply rubbing on oils or splashing on a watery liquid. It feels nicer and lasts longer.

An emulsion is rendered possible by the presence of an emulsifier, or sometimes more than one. Various emulsifiers are used in Nature's Way products: triethanolamine stearate is a liquid soap used in some cleansing lotions; nonionic emulsifiers are neutral materials often used at acid pH. All are large molecules with a hydrophilic head and a lipophilic tail.

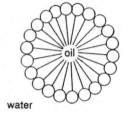

stylised representation of a single molecule of an emulsifier, showing a large polar (water-soluble) head and a long hydrocarbon (oil-soluble) chain

oil-in-water emulsion: molecules are orientated in clusters (micelles) so that the polar head is outermost and in the water phase

water

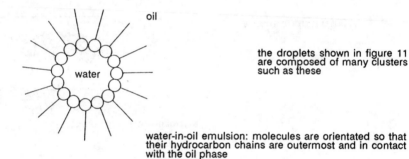

oil

water

the droplets shown in figure 11 are composed of many clusters such as these

water-in-oil emulsion: molecules are orientated so that their hydrocarbon chains are outermost and in contact with the oil phase

Figure 12. Structure of an emulsifier (diagrammatic)

Erythema. A medical term meaning reddening of the skin. When in response to sunlight it is the first stage of sunburn. It may also be in response to physical action or to chemical stimulation. Other causes range from viral and fungal infections to emotional blushing and the hot flushes of the menopause.

Essential Oils. The volatile oils, mainly from flowering plants, that are responsible for its fragrance. They contain ethers, alcohols and phenolic compounds as well as aldehydes, ketones and esters. They are named after their plant of origin and most are made up from many, many constituents. Because of their volatility and small molecular size they are readily absorbed through the epidermis and may even penetrate into the blood stream. They have long been used in perfumery, and the resurgence of interest in their therapeutic powers has led to the current popularity of aromatherapy.

Esters. The result of reacting a fatty acid with an alcohol, esters are much used in skin care for their spreading properties and "dry" oiliness. They reduce the greasy feel of mineral and vegetable oils, giving a lighter, more pleasant skin-feel and they often improve skin-penetrating properties because of their solvent powers, allowing them access through the epidermis by intercellular absorption. Many are available and different ones are selected for their differing effects.

Ethanol. Obtained by fermentation, ethanol is the alcohol present in wines and spirits but unfortunately without the pleasant taste. Small quantities are used in skin toners to speed evaporation and give a cooling effect. It has a slightly astringent action and, in the concentrations used, should not have a drying effect on skin. It is present in witch hazel as usually sold; for the Aloe Vera Toner and the Eye Gel a special alcohol-free witch hazel was commissioned.

Ethoxylation. If an oil is treated with ethylene oxide it can be rendered water-soluble and is said to be ethoxylated. This process is applied to many insoluble materials to produce soluble emollients and emulsifiers. The process can be carefully controlled to attain the specific degree of ethoxylation required to achieve the precise level of solubility desired.

The ethoxylated oil retains many of the emollient properties of the original. Products with a high degree of ethoxylation are very useful as solubilisers for perfume and other oils that are introduced into an aqueous or aqueous-alcoholic system.

Fragrance. As far as practicable, Nature's Way ranges use essential oils and natural fragrances. Fragrance-free products were offered but were not popular, so tried and tested fragrances are utilised where required.

Free Radicals. These are highly reactive atoms or molecules that are capable of initiating a chain reaction with stable molecules to generate more free radicals. This mechanism, which occurs in proteins and nucleic acids, can be enzyme-produced or photo (light)-induced. The result is damaged connective tissue which in turn results in a loss of elasticity and moisture-holding capacity of the skin leading to dryness and wrinkle formation.

Advances in products today are due to a better understanding of cause and effect. Thus, although we all knew that areas exposed to the sun looked older than skin that was not so exposed, it is only recently that the free-radical theory of ageing has been postulated and largely accepted. Now that there is an acceptable theory of ageing, products can be devised to prevent it, or at least delay the outward signs.

One way is to apply a free-radical scavenger to the skin via topical application. A free-radical scavenger works by preferentially reacting with the free radical, thus preventing it from reacting with dermal proteins. It also halts the chain reaction and further free-radical formation. (See also Vitamin E and UV Light.)

Glycerine. A common ingredient in emulsions and skin toners, it has moisture-holding properties which prevent products from drying out and which also help maintain the moisture balance in the skin. Because of its strong affinity for moisture, too much glycerine can actually dehydrate the skin. It can be of either animal or vegetable origin, being a by-product of soap production. Nature's Way only uses that from vegetable sources despite the price premium. (See Humectants.)

Glyceryl Stearate. Used extensively as an emulsifier and to give body to a cream without its feeling heavy. The glyceryl esters are formed by reacting glycerine, which is a polyhydric alcohol, with the relevant fatty acid. Because the acid is of natural origin it is a mixture of several acids and the resultant ester is a complex mixture. Glyceryl stearates vary considerably from different suppliers and they are also often treated to improve their value as an emulsifier. Nature's Way actually uses three different glyceryl stearates to achieve the results required in individual products.

Grape Seed Oil. Obtained from the seeds of muscat raisins. Over 50% of the oil is linoleic acid and it is therefore a useful source of vitamin F. It has little odour and is nearly colourless, which makes it useful for skin-care products. It is much used in massage and cleansing products, having a light and pleasant skin-feel, and as a carrier oil in aromatherapy.

Herbal Extracts. Obtained from the natural plant by various means — solvent extraction, steaming, boiling in water, etc. Different methods extract differing constituents; Nature's Way products utilise extracts that have not been obtained using glycols or ethanol as the extracting solvent. The extracts used are from plants which historical usage has proven to be of value in treating skin disorders or to have other beneficial effects.

Humectants. A humectant is a hygroscopic material, that is, one that has a strong affinity for water. Glycerine is perhaps the best known: a saucer of glycerine in the open air will attract moisture until it becomes quite diluted. If 5 to 10% glycerine is included in a cosmetic emulsion, it will prevent evaporation of the aqueous phase. When the product is applied to the skin it adheres to the epidermis and will hold water to it. However, 15% glycerine and above will absorb water from the skin, thus having a dehydrating effect.

Hydroxyoctacosanyl Hydroxystearate. A synthetic wax recommended as a consistency regulator for water-in-oil emulsions. It is claimed to improve skin-feel and the stability of pigmented products.

Interstitial. An interstice is a small space between things closely set. Thus the interstitial lipid film is the oily film between cells.

Iron oxide pigments. The famous coloured sands of Alum Bay, Isle of Wight, are due to traces of iron oxides in combination with other metallic salts. The iron oxide pigments used in cosmetics are synthesised to achieve the high standards of purity required for materials that come into contact with human skin. They are insoluble and very safe in use.

Isopropyl Myristate. An ester (q.v.).

Isopropyl Palmitate. An ester (q.v.).

Isostearyl Alcohol. Stearyl alcohol is a waxy solid but the *iso* form is a mobile liquid with emollient and superfatting properties.

Kaolin. A well-known cosmetic ingredient, it is a naturally occurring hydrated aluminium silicate found especially in Cornwall and is commonly known as china clay. Cosmetic grades are obtained by suspending the clay in water containing an electrolyte which keeps the fine particles in suspension. These are separated and the charge neutralised. It does not have the thickening power of bentonite, but is absorbent and is commonly used in face packs to absorb perspiration and sebum deposits.

Lactic Acid. Obtained by fermentation of starch or of lactose from creameries. A mild, naturally derived acid much used for adjusting the pH of cosmetics. In Nature's Way products it is usually used in conjunction with sodium lactate (q.v.).

Lanolin. Whilst not present in Nature's Way ranges as such, its derivatives are valuable constituents of some products. For fifty years lanolin was one of the most common of all skin-care ingredients, prized for its emollient and skin-softening properties. It is the sebum exuded by sheep onto their wool, which renders it waterproof, and which is collected from wool-combers as part of the wool-cleaning process. Unfortunately, in the late fifties some people developed allergies to insecticide residues from the sheep dip and later to strong surfactant residues used in the cleaning process. These materials are now removed by superior purifying techniques. Lanolin is composed of:

Fatty acids

Aliphatic acids	30.0%
Hydroxy acids	17.0
Cyclic acids	2.0
Unsaturated acids	2.0
subtotal	51.0%

Alcohols

Lanosterol	22.0%
Cholesterol	16.0
Monohydric alcohols	5.0
α- and β-diols	3.0
Agnosterol	1.0
subtotal	47.0%
minor constituents	to 100.0%

Lanolin Oil. Lanolin is a semi-hard, waxy solid which is difficult to handle. It can be separated into its constituent parts by low-temperature fractional crystallisation. The constituents that are solid at room temperature are removed and there remains a complex mixture of natural fatty acids, esters and alcohols, particularly cholesterol. It has not undergone chemical modification but is no longer lanolin in its entirety. It is an amber fluid which is easy to handle and which retains the water-in-oil emulsifying properties of the original material and all its emolliency and skin-moisturising properties.

Lauryl Betaine. An amphoteric surfactant used because of its mildness and ability to reduce potential irritation of other surfactants.

Lemon Juice. Historically, lemon juice has been used for cleaning and bleaching the skin. These properties are no doubt due to its citric acid content.

Lipid. Oil, often used as a generic name for the skin's own oil content.

Magnesium Aluminium Silicate. A swelling clay mined in Wyoming, USA. Clay is defined as a sedimentary deposit that has plastic properties when wet and that hardens and cracks when dry. It is composed of fine rock particles of less than 0.004 mm in diameter. Clays are thus mineral deposits and principally consist of hydrous silicates of magnesium and aluminium that occur as crystals with a layered structure capable of absorbing and losing water. There are vast deposits of clay throughout the world and because they are of natural origin different deposits have different compositions and differing properties.

Magnesium Sulphate. Commonly known as Epsom salts, it is used to stabilise water-in-oil emulsions.

Menthol. Naturally occurring in peppermint oil. When a dilute solution is applied to the skin, it produces vasodilation followed by a feeling of numbness and mild local anaesthesia due, it is believed, to differential stimulation of the sensory nerve endings[11].

Methoxy PEG-22/Dodecyl Glycol Copolymer. A nonionic water-in-oil emulsifier that is stable in the presence of electrolytes and over a wide pH range. It is claimed to be a good wetting agent for pigments and has excellent dermatological properties.

Methylchloroisothazolinone. A preservative (q.v.).

Methylparaben. A preservative (q.v.).

Methylsilanol Mannuronate. An organic silicon compound containing the mannuronate ion, a natural polysaccharide extracted from seaweed. It was developed in France specifically to have an anticellulite action. It is well documented and test results show its high penetrating powers, its lipolytic action and its cytostimulating action.

Milia. Hard white spots, usually found on the upper cheeks and eye area. The cause is a concentration of keratinised sebum below the skin, often blocking a sweat duct.

Mineral Oil. Also known as white oil and liquid paraffin; when pure grades became available, they largely superseded natural oils in cosmetics because of their cheapness and ease of use. It is described as "inert, inexpensive, safe, easily emulsified and functional".[12] Now, with the renewed interest in natural oils and greater expectations of a product's efficacy, mineral oil has been replaced in many products by natural oils and esters.

It still has a place in massage creams and oils, where its oiliness and non-penetrating properties are an advantage.

Mucopolysaccharides. These high-molecular-weight polymers are present throughout the animal kingdom, from bacteria to mammals. They are normally associated with proteins such as collagen, with which they are strongly bonded. They occur throughout the body in the skin, the bones and particularly in cartilage, where they have a lubricating action.

Although mucopolysaccharides are present in different forms in various areas of the body, they are all characterised by high molecular weights and they form highly viscous, even gelatinous, solutions which are slippery and sticky and strongly hydrophilic. They are present in high concentration in the dermis where the collagen and elastin fibres are embedded in a jelly of mucopolysaccharides.

Mucopolysaccharides are anionic and have a strong affinity for sodium, potassium and calcium ions, and this, coupled with their high degree of hydration, explains their role in maintaining the water and electrolyte properties of the skin. The mucopolysaccharides content of the dermis decreases with advancing age: there is a sharp decrease during the first ten years of life, followed by a slow decline until the mid-forties and then a steady reduction leading to dry and wrinkled skin.

As well as their hydrating properties, mucopolysaccharides appear to play an important part in wound-healing; it is suggested that this is because of their association with collagen, causing reticulation and fibrillation of this protein, and a higher than normal concentration of mucopolysaccharides is found in wound areas.

Because of their highly polar character they are very hydrophilic and have a great capacity to retain moisture.

Altogether, mucopolysaccharides play a very important part in maintaining the moisture content, texture and elasticity of skin. As their concentration decreases with age, the effects become apparent as a loss of skin tone and dryness.

Natural Moisturising Factor, or **NMF.** This is a complex mixture that exists in the stratum corneum and, in association with the lipid film from sebum, is emulsified into a water-in-oil emulsion by the cholesterol present. The NMF consists predominantly of:

Free amino acids   40.0%
Pyrrolidone carboxylic acid
(mostly as the sodium salt) 12.0%
Urea   7.0%
Lactic acid
(mostly as sodium lactate) 12.0%
Mineral salts, etc.   to 100.0%

Both sodium salts are strongly hygroscopic with a capacity to absorb water which is greater than glycerine, propylene glycol and sorbitol. The NMF is responsible for maintaining the moisture level in the epidermis.

Nonionic. See under Surfactants.

Octyl Palmitate. An ester (q.v.).

Oils, Fats and **Waxes.** An oil may be of animal or vegetable origin or be synthetic. All natural oils consist of fatty acids and fatty acid glycerides. This means that the naturally occurring fatty acid has reacted with glycerine to give the glyceryl ester. The fatty acids are so called because they are commonly found in fats.

Oils, fats and waxes do not mix with water. An oil is liquid at room temperature, a fat is a pasty solid and a wax is hard and often brittle. A fat contains mostly saturated fatty acids and is normally of animal origin; an oil contains mostly unsaturated fatty acids and is usually of plant origin.

Oleyl Alcohol. An oily liquid, it is used in place of cetearyl alcohol where a softer, less viscous product is required. It has good solvent properties for oil-based grime, so is useful in cleansing preparations.

Paraffin Wax. Paraffin wax is a mixture of hard hydrocarbons obtained from petroleum oils. It occurs as a white, crystalline, translucent mass with a greasy feel. Many grades are available, differentiated by their melting points but all within the range of 42°C to 65°C.

PEG-6 Caprylic/Capric Triglyceride. The ethoxylated form of caprylic/capric triglyceride, which make this oil partially soluble in water. The oiliness it imparts to aqueous products gives them refatting properties. An unfortunate side-effect of bathing, especially if in a bubble bath, is drying of the skin, because warm water leeches out essential protective oils from the epidermis and possibly the dermis. PEG-6 caprylic/capric triglyceride is a refatting agent which is incorporated with aloe vera gel in the Enriched Foaming Bath Oil. Tests in Germany showed that using this material in a bath twice weekly was beneficial to patients with deficient sebaceous gland secretions and subjects with endogenous eczema and *ichthyosis vulgaris*. It was seen that skin dryness regressed considerably and the non-irritating effect of the baths on the skin of eczematous patients was particularly noteworthy.

However, it is not necessary to have any of these skin complaints to enjoy a Nature's Way Enriched Foam Bath; just relax in its soft, fragrant bubbles and enjoy it with confidence.

PEG-150 Distearate. A waxy solid, soluble in water, used to thicken surfactant-based products. It improves the skin-feel of such products and reduces the irritation potential of foaming agents.

PEG-45/Dodecyl Glycol Copolymer. Claimed to be a good water-in-oil emulsion stabiliser and to be of particular use in pigmented products, where it aids pigment wetting, dispersion and suspension as well as improving emolliency and spreading properties.

PEG-60 Hydrogenated Castor Oil. A nonionic surfactant (q.v.), used as a solubiliser to clarify skin toners.

Pentaerythritol. A water-in-oil emulsifier (q.v.).

Petrolatum. Also known as petroleum jelly, it is another hydrocarbon from the petroleum industry with cosmetic applications, familiar to us all as Vaseline. Like mineral oil and the hydrocarbon waxes, it is a common constituent of emulsion products, especially where a film is required on the skin's surface. None of the hydrocarbons are absorbed by the skin and the texture of products made with them tends to feel heavy and can drag on application.

pH. Not an ingredient but a measure of acidity and alkalinity, measured on a scale of 1 to 14. Below pH 7 is acid, pH 7 is neutral and above 7 is alkaline.

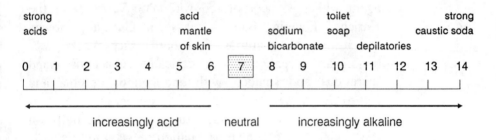

Figure 13. pH scale

There are two different reasons why pH is important to skin-care products: the pH matters because of the intended use of the product and also because the pH can affect the product's stability.

There are valid reasons for formulating certain products to match the pH of the skin; however, others are best at a neutral or alkaline pH. It is generally accepted that cleansers should be neutral to slightly alkaline, toners and fresheners should be acid, and moisturisers and night creams may be between pH 5 and 7.5. However, certain active ingredients may require higher or lower values to be effective, and products will be adjusted accordingly. Astringents are usually acid; cationic materials that are used both as emulsifiers and bactericides need to be at an acid pH. Triethanolamine stearate emulsions are slightly alkaline; carbomer gels need to be above pH 6.5 for maximum gel strength; depilatories have a pH of 11+; soaps are normally at pH 10. Acne creams are usually from pH 5 to 5.5 and most preservatives and bactericides are more effective at an acid pH. Blood and tears are slightly alkaline and eye products are usually made neutral for minimum irritancy.

Many colours are affected by pH changes and herbal extracts may precipitate organic matter at an acid or alkaline pH. Panthenol, which is used extensively in hair and skin products, is stable between pH 4 and 6, and protein materials and unsaturated fatty acids are best applied at a slightly acid pH. So although not an ingredient, pH is one of the most important properties of any skin-care product.[4]

Phosphoric Acid. Used to adjust pH (q.v.) in products where lactic acid is not suitable.

Polar. A polar molecule is defined as one in which the electrons forming the valency bond are not symmetrically arranged. In practice, this includes water and ethanol as highly polar substances; mineral oil is non-polar. Polar materials are often good solvents and are themselves usually soluble in water, whereas non-polar materials are oil-soluble. However, many oily, water-insoluble, substances, including many vegetable oils, triglycerides and esters, are also polar.

The cosmetic advantage of polar oils is that they spread readily on the skin, are excellent cleansers for oil-based grime and they do not clog pores. Non-polar oils have good barrier properties and are useful where an extended application time is required or where an occlusive film will improve skin hydration.

Polawax. A proprietary emulsifier (q.v.). The manufacturers refuse to divulge the material content of this emulsifier, but it is of vegetable origin and has a very long history of satisfactory use in skin-care products.

Polyethoxylated (150) Lanolin. Obtained by ethoxylation (q.v.) of lanolin. The ethoxylated material retains many of the emollient properties of lanolin. It is used to reduce the harshness of surfactant-based systems and is claimed to have a refatting action.

Polyglycerylmethacrylate. This material has been developed as a surgical lubricant, and extensive testing on human volunteers has proved its safety. It is a non-drying gel which retains its physical characteristics even when incorporated in a cosmetic product. It is deposited on the skin as a monomolecular film which gives the skin a smooth silky feel. 98% of its gel structure is water of hydration which is held in contact with the skin, and it thus acts as a beneficial moisturiser.

Polysorbate 20. A nonionic emulsifier (q.v.).

Polysorbate 40. A nonionic emulsifier (q.v.).

Polyvinylpyrrolidone. Commonly known as PVP, it is a film-forming polymer. It is used in a hydrating mask to strengthen the occlusive film on the skin. It is substantive to skin and leaves it feeling soft and smooth. Because it is hygroscopic it also acts as a moisturising agent.

Preservatives. Unfortunately bacteria and fungal spores are ubiquitous, and cosmetic and toiletry products are often an attractive medium in which they can multiply, which they do at a phenomenal rate, approximately doubling in numbers every twenty minutes under ideal conditions. Even products that have been properly formulated and carefully made can still become contaminated in use or during storage, so a preservative is introduced to control bacterial growth.

By their very nature, preservatives have to be toxic, so in cases of allergy they are always high on the list of suspects. One preservative cannot be used for all products as some only work over a narrow pH-range, while others may be inactivated by the materials in the product. Care is taken to use the minimal quantity required to reduce the risk of allergy and frequently two or more different ones are used to provide the broad spectrum of safety required without using an unacceptably high level of any one particular preservative.

Propylparaben. A preservative (q.v.).

Propylene Glycol. Much used as a humectant (q.v.). Its action is similar to that of glycerine and it also has some antifungal activity against skin flora.

Propylene Glycol Dicaprylate. A light emollient oil.

Propylene Phenoxytol. A preservative which also has bactericidal properties against the bacteria associated with skin infections.

Proteins. Proteins are the basis of life. Relatively simple amino acids combine together in a pre-set order to form a peptide chain, the bonding process being controlled by the organism's chromosomes. The result is all the various forms of protein in the body. From the keratin of nails and hair to the flesh of muscles and internal organs, all are composed of amino acids in combination to form specific proteins.

Rosemary Oil. An essential oil (q.v.) with good bactericidal properties and a pleasant, fresh odour. See chapter 5 on aromatherapy for more details.

Rubefacient. A rubefacient has a warming effect when applied to skin, which it achieves by causing a slight irritation that produces a histological reaction plus vasodilation of the blood vessels. Rubefacients stimulate dermal activity and are useful in hydrating masks.

Saponification. The reaction between an alkali and a fatty acid to form a soap and glycerine. The physical characteristics of the soap depend on the fatty acids and alkali used; triethanolamine gives a liquid soap, potassium hydroxide a soft one and sodium hydroxide a hard soap. Fatty acids of vegetable origin produce softer soaps than those derived from animal tallow.

Sodium Borate. Commonly known as borax, it is a mild alkali which is used in conjunction with beeswax to form an emulsion. The borax saponifies the beeswax fatty acids to form a soap which then acts as an emulsifier.

Sodium Chloride. An electrolyte, familiar as common salt.

Sodium Hydroxide. Commonly known as caustic soda, it is used to neutralise acidic materials and to saponify fatty acids in soap production.

Sodium Lactate. The salt of lactic acid, it is used in association with the acid to form a buffer solution at pH 5.3 to 5.5, which matches the natural acid mantle of the skin. (See also Lactic Acid, pH, Acid Mantle, Buffers and Natural Moisturising Factor, or NMF.)

Sodium Laureth Sulphate. An anionic surfactant (see under Surfactants).

Sodium Lauryl Sulphate. An anionic surfactant used at low concentration as an emulsifier.

Sodium PCA. The sodium salt of pyrrolidone carboxylic acid, it is a moisturising agent and an essential constituent of the acid mantle (q.v.) of the skin.

Soluble Colours. Life would be extremely dull without colour and although the colour of the majority of Nature's Way products is natural, now and again we could not resist improving upon nature by adding a little soluble colour.

Colours can be named in a variety of ways. Universally they have a Colour Index number, shown as "C.I." followed by a multidigit number. In the United States and many parts of the world they are listed as "FD & C" or "D & C" followed by a one- or two-digit number. FD & C means passed for use in food, drugs and cosmetics, D & C for use in drugs and cosmetics only. Soluble colours also have trivial names such as Sunset Yellow, Alizarin, Tartrazine, etc. Finally, they may have "E" numbers awarded by the European Community.

In the Nature's Way ingredient listing colours are shown using the (F)D & C system. In the following table they are listed by their C.I. numbers, their E numbers, where applicable, and their trivial names. All have been passed for use in cosmetics in both America and Europe, provided that the batches of dyestuff are tested before release and meet the specification of the relevant governing body.

	Trivial Name	C.I. No.	E No.
D & C Red No. 33		17200	
D & C Yellow No. 8	Uranine	45350	
D & C Yellow No. 10	Quinoline Yellow	47005	E 104
FD & C Blue No. 1	Brilliant Blue FCF	42090	E 133
FD & C Yellow No. 5	Tartrazine	19140	E 102
FD & C Yellow No. 6	Sunset Yellow	15985	E 110

Sorbitan Oleate. A nonionic emulsifier (q.v.).

Sorbitan Palmitate. A nonionic emulsifier (q.v.).

Stearic Acid. One of the most common of all skin-care emulsion ingredients, it can be of either animal or vegetable origin although only that from vegetable sources is used in Nature's Way products. It is a white, waxy solid which is often saponified *in situ* by triethanolamine (q.v.) to form an oil-in-water emulsifier. Because it is a soft soap it is excellent as the emulsifier in cleansing lotions. Stearic acid is not always saponified in emulsions; as an ingredient of the oil phase it crystallises to give a pearly sheen to the product and a "dry" emollience to the skin.

Sulphur Tar Complex. Coal-tar extract was long used as an anti-acne and antidandruff agent but because of adulterants such as toluene, benzene, cresols, etc. it is no longer thought suitable for topical application. The sulphur tar complex used in Nature's Way Chamomile Toner fulfils the original function of coal-tar extract without any of the unwelcome contaminants.

Sulphur tar complex is extracted from willow oleoresin and is dermatologically excellent for the topical treatment of skin diseases.

Surfactants. *Surfactant* is a simplified term for surface-active agent. A surface-active agent is one which affects the surface tension of a liquid. Emulsifiers and detergents are surfactants: by reducing the surface tension of water they reduce its tendency to form droplets and make it spread more easily.

Surfactant molecules consist of two parts, a hydrophilic head which is water-soluble and a lipophilic tail which is oil-soluble (see under Emulsifiers). Surfactants are divided into four categories: anionic, cationic, amphoteric and nonionic. This classification depends on whether they ionise in solution (i.e., form electrically charged groups) and the nature of the predominant ion.

Anionic surfactants are the salts of a strong acid, such as sulphuric acid, which renders the normally lipophilic tail water-soluble, so that the surfactant will readily emulsify oil into water, making the material a good cleaning agent and emulsifier.

Cationic surfactants are quaternary ammonium compounds. The cation is the water-soluble part responsible for reducing surface activity. Cationic surfactants are poor cleansers but are substantive to keratin, making them good conditioning agents; they are also bactericidal.

Amphoteric surfactants are more ionically in balance than the anionic and cationic surfactants: they ionise according to the pH of the solution. Generally they are poor emulsifiers but work well in combination with anionic surfactants, boosting foaming properties and reducing irritation.

Nonionic surfactants do not ionise in water and are poor cleansing and foaming agents, but when selected with care they make excellent emulsifiers, little affected by the product's pH, and stable in the presence of electrolytes.

Titanium Dioxide. Of all the natural hazards to which skin is exposed, potentially the most damaging is sunlight. Chemical sun-screens have long been used to achieve a tan without sunburn but now it has been found that all ultraviolet light (see UV light) is potentially harmful and a broad sun-screen filter is required.

To achieve this broad-spectrum protection without an unacceptable level of reactive chemical sun-filters, a microfine titanium dioxide has been devised which reflects sunlight without a whitening effect on the skin. This is incorporated in both the Aloe Vera Moisturiser and Night Cream as many people use the latter product when sailing or skiing, when extra protection is required. For greater protection, there are two sun-protection products, one at sun-protection factor (SPF) 14, the other at SPF 25+.

Triethanolamine. A relatively mild alkali used to saponify stearic acid to form the emulsifier triethanolamine stearate.

Triglycerides. Frequently referred to in association with other materials, a triglyceride results when the three hydroxyl (-OH) groups of glycerine are replaced with the hydrocarbon chains of fatty acids.

UV Light. Ultraviolet light — electromagnetic radiation in the range of 4-400 nanometers.

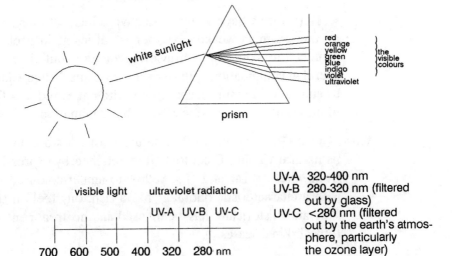

Figure 14. Light wavelengths

Areas of skin exposed to the sun age quicker than skin that is not so exposed. One reason is that the ultraviolet light causes the formation of free radicals (q.v.) within the skin, leading to damaged connective tissue. There is a consequent loss of elasticity and moisture-holding capacity and the results are dryness and wrinkle formation.

Until very recently, sun-screen products were designed to stop the UV-B light responsible for erythema while allowing the maximum amount of UV-A light, which is responsible for sun-tanning, to reach the skin. Now it has been proven that UV-A light is as damaging as UV-B and is responsible for skin cancers as well as hastening the ageing process. See also Titanium Dioxide.

Vegetable Oil. Usually soya oil, used in massage creams and other creams where an oily feel and an extended application time are required.

Vitamin E. This is d-α-tocopheryl acetate and less prone to oxidation than *d*-α-tocopherol. The latter is used as a natural antioxidant and is the only truly natural antioxidant to be used in food. If the acetate is used in a skin preparation it breaks down to the antioxidant form and becomes a free radical scavenger (see Free Radicals).

Both forms have a sun-protective effect, although the acetate is much weaker. Neither is sufficient in itself to protect the skin from ultraviolet radiation but they are useful in combination with sun-screen agents. When added to sun and after-sun preparations, vitamin E reduces the redness and swelling associated with inflammation.

Wheat Germ Oil. A popular oil in natural cosmetics because of its natural vitamin E content. It is obtained by expression from wheat germ and is a yellow-to-amber-coloured oil with a characteristic odour. It has a rich, oily feel on the skin and historically has been used in the treatment of topical skin diseases.

Witch Hazel. Also known as hamamelis water and extracted from the leaves and bark of the bush *Hamamelis virginiana*. The extract is distilled to remove much of the tannin and it contains approximately 13% ethanol. It is well known as a mild astringent and a soothing and healing agent, largely due to its essential oil containing carvacrol, eugenol, safrole, hexanol and sesquiterpene alcohols, which also exert a mild disinfecting action.

Witch Hazel Special. To avoid the ethanol content of regular witch hazel, a special extract was commissioned for the Aloe Vera Toner and Eye Gel.

Wool Wax Alcohols. A derivative of lanolin (q.v.), pure lanolin is treated with potassium hydroxide until it is saponified. The result can be separated into wool wax alcohols and lanolin fatty acids. Wool wax alcohols are useful as water-in-oil emulsifiers, their emulsifying action being due to the cholesterol content. Cholesterol is a major constituent in human sebum so its use in cosmetics and pharmaceutical creams has long been popular. Interestingly, in the 1930s, cholesterol was advocated as a hair restorer. Although its efficacy as such a remedy was later disproved, it may account for the belief that lanolin caused hair growth.

Xanthan Gum. Much used by the food industry, it is becoming popular in cosmetics. It comes from fermented corn starch and is a polysaccharide salt. It is easier to disperse than many of the gums, and the viscosity of products thickened with xanthan gum is almost independent of temperature.

Zinc Oxide. An insoluble white powder with a mildly astringent action, making it popular in soothing preparations including products for a greasy skin. It is very white and was long used as a constituent of face powders. However, titanium dioxide has much greater opacity and whiteness and has largely replaced it in such products.

Chapter Nine

Nature's Way Ingredient Listing

Below is a complete list of all Nature's Way products and a full disclosure of their ingredients at the time of going to press. It is inevitable that in such a dynamic range of products as Nature's Way's occasional changes in composition will be made. Bellitas Limited, the manufacturers and distributors of Nature's Way, periodically publish a newsletter which gives details of any formula changes, as well as hints and tips on treatments and details of special offers on Nature's Way and other Bellitas skin-care products. To receive your free copy of the newsletter, simply drop a line on your business notepaper to Bellitas; their address is at the front of the book.

The products are arranged in the list according to their type. Against each product is a reference number, the pH value, a letter denoting the COSHH group to which it belongs and the pack sizes available. The pH value is the mid-point of the product's specification and the reference number will enable you to identify the formula should you have any queries about the product. The COSHH group letter refers to essential health and safety data, details of which appear in chapter 10.

Chamomile for Oily and Problem Skin

Chamomile Face Wash   Ref. BT 0429

COSHH Group E   pH 5.3

Essential Oil of Chamomile, FD & C Blue No. 1, Lauryl
Betaine, PEG-150 Distearate, Phosphoric Acid,
Propylene Phenoxytol, Sodium Laureth Sulphate, Water.

Available in 200 ml bottles

Chamomile Mask   Ref. BT 0099

COSHH Group A   pH 5.3

Dichlorobenzyl Alcohol, Essential Oil of Chamomile,
Iron Oxide Pigments, Kaolin, Lactic Acid, Magnesium
Aluminium Silicate, Polyglycerylmethacrylate, Propylene
Glycol, Propylene Phenoxytol, Sodium Lactate, Sulphur
Tar Complex, Xanthan Gum, Water.

Sizes available: 50 g and 365 g jars

Chamomile Toner   Ref. BT 0371

COSHH Group B   pH 5.3

Denatonium Benzoate, Essential Oil of Chamomile,
Essential Oil of Rosemary, Ethanol, FD & C Yellow No.
5, Lactic Acid, Polysorbate 20, Propylene Glycol,
Propylene Phenoxytol, Sodium Lactate, Sulphur Tar
Complex, Witch Hazel BPC, Water. .

Available in 200 ml bottles

Chamomile Moisturiser Lotion   Ref. BT 0384

COSHH Group A   pH 5.3

Almond Oil (Sweet), BHA, Caprylic/Capric Triglyceride,
Cocoa Butter, DEA-Oleth-3 Phosphate, Essential Oil of
Chamomile, Iron Oxide Pigments, Lactic Acid, Methyl-

paraben, Polawax (vegetable source), Propylene Glycol, Propylparaben, Sodium Lactate, Sodium PCA, Xanthan Gum, Zinc Oxide, Water.

Available in 200 ml bottles

Natural Range for Oily to Normal Skin

Grapefruit Wash-off Cleansing Gel   Ref. BT 0107

COSHH Group E   pH 7.3

Cocoamphocarboxyglycinate, D & C Yellow No. 10, Grapefruit Juice, Grapefruit Oil, Methylchloroiso- thiazolinone, PEG-150 Distearate, Sodium Laureth Sulphate, Water.

Packed in a handy 100 ml tube

Peach Deep Cleansing Mask   Ref. BT 0105

COSHH Group A   pH 7.5

Beeswax, Cetearyl Alcohol, DEA-Oleth-3 Phosphate, Dichlorobenzyl Alcohol, Fragrance, Iron Oxide Pigments, Kaolin, Magnesium Aluminium Silicate, Methylchloroiso- thiazolinone, Peach Kernel Oil, Propylene Glycol, Xanthan Gum, Zinc Oxide, Water.

Sizes available: 50 g and 365 g jars

Lemon Cleansing Lotion   Ref. BT 0351

COSHH Group A   pH 7.5

BHA, Carbomer, Cetearyl Alcohol, D & C Yellow No. 8, D & C Yellow No. 10, EDTA Disodium Salt, Fragrance, Glyceryl Stearate, Methylchloroisothiazolinone, Mineral Oil, Oleyl Alcohol, Polysorbate 20, Pure Lemon Juice, Stearic Acid, Triethanolamine, Water.

Sizes available: 200 ml and 500 ml bottles

Cucumber Toner   Ref. BT 0367

COSHH Group B   pH 5.3

Cucumber Extract, Denatonium Benzoate, Ethanol, FD
& C Blue No. 1, FD & C Yellow No. 5, Fragrance,
Glycerine, PEG-60 Hydrogenated Castor Oil, Sodium
Lactate, Witch Hazel BPC, Water.

Sizes available: 200 ml and 500 ml bottles

Avocado Day Moisturiser   Ref. BT 0378

COSHH Group A   pH 5.3

Acetylated Lanolin Alcohol, Almond Oil (Sweet),
Avocado Oil, Beeswax, BHA, Caprylic/Capric Tri-
glyceride, Cocoa Butter, Dichlorobenzyl Alcohol, FD & C
Blue No. 1, FD & C Yellow No. 5, Fragrance, Glycerine,
Glyceryl Stearate, Methylchloroisothiazolinone, Polawax
(vegetable source), Propylene Glycol Dicaprylate,
Propylparaben, Sodium Lactate, Water.

Sizes available: 50 g and 365 g jars

Ginseng for Normal to Dry Skin

Ginseng Stimulating Mask   Ref. BT 0102

COSHH Group A   pH 5.5

Almond Oil (Sweet), BHA, Ceteareth-20, Cetearyl
Alcohol, Cocoa Butter, Dichlorobenzyl Alcohol,
Dimethicone, D & C Yellow No. 6, Extract of Ginseng,
FD & C Yellow No. 5, Fragrance, Lactic Acid, Methyl-
chloroisothiazolinone, Polyglycerylmethacrylate,
Propylene Glycol, Sodium Lactate, Water.

Sizes available: 50 g and 365 g jars

Ginseng Cleanser   Ref. BT 0350

COSHH Group A   pH 7.5

BHA, Carbomer, Cetearyl Alcohol, D & C Yellow No. 6,
Extract of Ginseng, FD & C Yellow No. 5, Fragrance,
Glyceryl Stearate, Methylchloroisothiazolinone, Mineral
Oil, Oleyl Alcohol, Polysorbate 20, Stearic Acid,
Triethanolamine, Water.

Sizes available: 200 ml and 500 ml bottles

Ginseng Toner   Ref. BT 0366

COSHH Group B   pH 5.7

Denatonium Benzoate, D & C Yellow No. 6, Ethanol,
Extract of Ginseng, Fragrance, Glycerine, PEG-60
Hydrogenated Castor Oil, Sodium Lactate, Witch Hazel
BPC, Water.

Sizes available: 200 ml and 500 ml bottles

Ginseng Moisturiser   Ref. BT 0377

COSHH Group A   pH 7.6

BHA, Caprylic/Capric Triglyceride, D & C Yellow No. 6,
Dichlorobenzyl Alcohol, Extract of Ginseng, FD & C
Yellow No. 5, Fragrance, Glycerine, Glyceryl Stearate,
Methylchloroisothiazolinone, Oleyl Alcohol, Polawax
(vegetable source), Propylparaben, Stearic Acid,
Triethanolamine, Water.

Sizes available: 50 g and 365 g jars

Ginseng Night Cream   Ref. BT 0399

COSHH Group A   pH 7.3

Caprylic/Capric Triglyceride, Cetearyl Alcohol, D & C
Yellow No. 6, Dichlorobenzyl Alcohol, Extract of

Ginseng, FD & C Yellow No. 5, Fragrance, Methylchloro-isothiazolinone, Mineral Oil, Petrolatum, Propylene Glycol, Polysorbate 20, Sorbitan Palmitate, Sodium Borate, Stearic Acid, Water.

Available in 50 g jars

Aloe Vera for Delicate Skin

Aloe Vera Wash-off Cleansing Gel   Ref. BT 0108

COSHH Group E   pH 7.3

Aloe Vera Gel, Azulene, Cocoamphocarboxyglycinate, Essential Oil of Chamomile, Methylchloroisothiazolin-one, PEG-150 Distearate, Sodium Laureth Sulphate, Water.

Packed in a handy 100 ml tube

Aloe Vera Cleanser   Ref. BT 0348

COSHH Group A   pH 7.3

Almond Oil (Sweet), Aloe Vera Gel, BHA, Caprylic/Capric Triglyceride, Cetearyl Alcohol, EDTA Disodium Salt, Essential Oil of Chamomile, Glyceryl Stearate, Grapeseed Oil, Methylchloroisothiazolinone, Polysorbate 20, Stearic Acid, Triethanolamine, Xanthan Gum, Water.

Available in 200 ml bottles

Aloe Vera Toner   Ref. BT 0373

COSHH Group B   pH 5.3

Aloe Vera Gel, Azulene, Essential Oil of Chamomile, Lactic Acid, Methylchloroisothiazolinone, Propylene Glycol, Sodium Lactate, Witch Hazel (Special), Water.

Available in 200 ml bottles

Aloe Vera Moisturiser Ref. BT 0375

COSHH Group A pH 5.5

Almond Oil (Sweet), Aloe Vera Gel, Avocado Oil,
Beeswax, Caprylic/Capric Triglyceride, Cocoa Butter,
Dichlorobenzyl Alcohol, Dimethicone, Essential Oil of
Chamomile, Glyceryl Stearate, Lactic Acid, Methylchloro-
isothiazolinone, Polawax (vegetable source), Polyglyceryl-
methacrylate, Propylene Glycol, Sodium PCA, Titanium
Dioxide, Water.

Available in 50 g jars

Aloe Vera Night Cream Ref. BT 0398

COSHH Group A pH 5.5

Acetylated Lanolin Alcohol, Aloe Vera Gel,
Caprylic/Capric Triglyceride, Cetearyl Octanoate,
Dichlorobenzyl Alcohol, Dimethicone, Essential Oil of
Chamomile, Glyceryl Stearate, Methylchloroisothiazolin-
one, Propylparaben, Propylene Glycol, Stearic Acid,
Titanium Dioxide, Xanthan Gum, Water.

Available in 50 g jars

Aloe Vera Soothing Gel Mask Ref. BT 0104

COSHH Group A pH 7.3

Aloe Vera Gel, Azulene, Carbomer, Dichlorobenzyl
Alcohol, EDTA Disodium Salt, Essential Oil of
Chamomile, Glycerine, Methylchloroisothiazolinone,
Polyvinylpyrrolidone, Stearyl Heptonate, Triethanol-
amine, Witch Hazel BPC, Water.

Sizes available: 50 g and 365 g jars

Sweet Almond for Drier Skin

Sweet Almond Cleanser   Ref. BT 0353

COSHH Group A   pH 6.2

Almond Oil (Sweet), Beeswax, BHA, Caprylic/Capric
Triglyceride, D & C Red No. 33, Decyl Oleate, Fragrance,
Methylchloroisothiazolinone, Polysorbate 20, Sodium
Lactate, Sorbitan Palmitate, Xanthan Gum, Water.

Sizes available: 200 ml and 500 ml bottles

Sweet Almond Toner   Ref. BT 0369

COSHH Group B   pH 5.5

Denatonium Benzoate, D & C Yellow No. 6, D & C Red
No. 33, Ethanol, Fragrance of Almond Blossom,
Glycerine, PEG-60 Hydrogenated Castor Oil, Sodium
PCA, Witch Hazel BPC, Water.

Sizes available: 200 ml and 500 ml bottles

Sweet Almond Moisturiser   Ref. BT 0381

COSHH Group A   pH 5.3

Acetylated Lanolin Alcohol, Almond Oil (Sweet),
Avocado Oil, Beeswax, BHA, Caprylic/Capric
Triglyceride, Cocoa Butter, Dichlorobenzyl Alcohol,
Fragrance, Glycerine, Glyceryl Stearate, Methylchloro-
isothiazolinone, Polawax (vegetable source), Propylene
Glycol Dicaprylate, Propylparaben, Sodium PCA, Water.

Sizes available: 50 g and 365 g jars

Sweet Almond Night Cream   Ref. BT 0402

COSHH Group A   pH 7.3

Almond Oil (Sweet), Avocado Oil, Caprylic/Capric
Triglyceride, Cetearyl Alcohol, Dichlorobenzyl Alcohol,

Fragrance, Glyceryl Stearate, Grapeseed Oil, Methyl-
chloroisothiazolinone, Methylparaben, Propylene Glycol,
Sodium Lactate, Sodium PCA, Stearic Acid,
Triethanolamine, Vitamin E, Wheat Germ Oil, Water.

Available in 50 g jars

Sweet Almond Enriched Cream Mask   Ref. BT 0103

COSHH Group A   pH 5.5

Almond Oil (Sweet), BHA, Ceteareth-20, Cetearyl
Alcohol, Cocoa Butter, Dichlorobenzyl Alcohol,
Dimethicone, D & C Red No. 33, Fragrance, Glycerine,
Lactic Acid, Methylchloroisothiazolinone,
Polyglycerylmethacrylate, Sodium Lactate, Water.

Sizes available: 50 g and 365 g jars

Collagen for Dry and Mature Skin

Collagen Cleansing Lotion   Ref. BT 0354

COSHH Group A   pH 5.3

Almond Oil (Sweet), Beeswax, BHA, Caprylic/Capric
Triglyceride, Collagen (Hydrolysed Vegetable Protein),
Decyl Oleate, Geranium Oil, Lavender Oil, Magnesium
Aluminium Silicate, Methylchloroisothiazolinone,
Polysorbate 20, Sodium Lactate, Sorbitan Palmitate,
Xanthan Gum, Water.

Available in 200 ml bottles

Collagen Toner   Ref. BT 0370

COSHH Group B   pH 5.5

Collagen (Hydrolysed Vegetable Protein), Denatonium
Benzoate, D & C Yellow No. 6, Ethanol, FD & C Yellow
No. 5, Geranium Oil, Glycerine, Lactic Acid, Lavender

Oil, PEG-6 Caprylic/Capric Glyceride, Sodium PCA,
Witch Hazel BPC, Water.

Available in 200 ml bottles

Collagen Moisturiser   Ref. BT 0382

COSHH Group A   pH 4.8

Acetylated Lanolin Alcohol, Beeswax, BHA, Caprylic/
Capric Triglyceride, Cocoa Butter, Collagen (Hydrolysed
Vegetable Protein), Dichlorobenzyl Alcohol, Geranium
Oil, Glycerine, Glyceryl Stearate, Lavender Oil, Methyl-
chloroisothiazolinone, Propylene Glycol Dicaprylate,
Polawax (vegetable source), Propylparaben, Sodium
Lactate, Water.

Available in 50 g jars

Collagen Night Cream   Ref. BT 0403

COSHH Group A   pH 5.6

Beeswax, BHA, Caprylic/Capric Triglyceride, Cetearyl
Alcohol, Collagen (Hydrolysed Vegetable Protein),
Dichlorobenzyl Alcohol, EDTA Disodium Salt, Geranium
Oil, Hydroxyoctacosanyl Hydroxystearate, Isostearyl
Alcohol, Lactic Acid, Lanolin Oil, Lavender Oil,
Magnesium Sulphate, Methylparaben, Pentaerythritol,
PEG-45/Dodecyl Glycol Copolymer, Propylene Glycol,
Sodium PCA, Water.

Available in 50 g jars

Collagen Hydrating Mask   Ref. BT 0106

COSHH Group A   pH 6.3

Caprylic/Capric Triglyceride, Carbomer, Cetearyl Alcohol,
Cocoa Butter, Collagen (Hydrolysed Vegetable Protein),
Dichlorobenzyl Alcohol, Glyceryl Stearate, Lactic Acid,

Methylparaben, Propylene Glycol, Propylparaben, Rosemary Oil, Sodium PCA, Triethanolamine, Water.

Sizes available: 50 g and 365 g jars

For the Eyes

Eye Make-up Remover No. 1   Ref. BT 0360

COSHH Group C

Decyl Oleate, Mineral Oil, Octyl Palmitate.

Sizes available: 200 ml and 500 ml bottles

Eye Make-up Remover No. 2   Ref. BT 0361

COSHH Group E   pH 6.5

Cocoamphocarboxyglycinate, Methylparaben, PEG-150 Distearate, Water.

Sizes available: 200 ml and 500 ml bottles

Eye Make-up Remover Gel   Ref. BT 0362

COSHH Group C

Isopropyl Myristate, Mineral Oil, Silica.

Packed in a handy 100 ml tube

Eye Gel   Ref. BT 0410

COSHH Group A   pH 7.0

Carbomer, D & C Yellow No. 8, EDTA Disodium Salt, Extract of Chamomile, FD & C Blue No. 1, Glycerine, Methylparaben, Polyvinylpyrrolidone, Triethanolamine, Witch Hazel (Special), Water.

Available in 30 g glass jars

Eye Cream with Vitamin E   Ref. BT 0412

COSHH Group A   pH 5.6

Beeswax, BHA, Caprylic/Capric Triglyceride, Cetearyl
Alcohol, Collagen (Hydrolyzed Vegetable Protein),
Dichlorobenzyl Alcohol, EDTA Disodium Salt,
Hydroxyoctacosanyl Hydroxystearate, Isostearyl Alcohol,
Lactic Acid, Lanolin Oil, Magnesium Sulphate, Methoxy
PEG-22/Dodecyl Glycol Copolymer, Methylparaben,
Pentaerythritol, Propylene Glycol, PEG-45/Dodecyl
Glycol Copolymer, Sodium PCA, Vitamin E
(α-Tocopheryl Acetate), Water.

Available in 30 g glass jars

For the Body

Neck Cream with Vitamin E and Vegetable Collagen

Ref. BT 0405

COSHH Group A   pH 5.6

Beeswax, BHA, Caprylic/Capric Triglyceride, Cetearyl
Alcohol, Collagen (Hydrolyzed Vegetable Protein),
Dichlorobenzyl Alcohol, EDTA Disodium Salt, Geranium
Oil, Hydroxyoctacosanyl Hydroxystearate, Isostearyl
Alcohol, Lactic Acid, Lanolin Oil, Lavender Oil,
Magnesium Sulphate, Methoxy PEG-22/Dodecyl Glycol
Copolymer, Methylparaben, Pentaerythritol, Propylene
Glycol, PEG-45/Dodecyl Glycol Copolymer, Sodium
PCA, Vitamin E (α-Tocopheryl Acetate), Ylang-Ylang
Oil, Water.

Available in 30 g glass jars

Facial Scrub   Ref. BT 0430

COSHH Group E   pH 5.5

Aloe Vera Gel, Cocoamphocarboxyglycinate, Exfolients,
Lavender Oil, Methylchloroisothiazolinone, PEG-150
Distearate, Sodium Laureth Sulphate, Water.

Packed in a handy 100 ml tube

Body Scrub   Ref. BT 0432

COSHH Group A   pH 7.8

Almond Oil (Sweet), BHA, Cetearyl Alcohol, Dichloro-
benzyl Alcohol, Exfolients, Iron Oxide Pigments,
Lavender Oil, Magnesium Aluminium Silicate, Methyl-
chloroisothiazolinone, Oleyl Alcohol, Propylene Glycol,
Sodium Lauryl Sulphate, Soybean Oil, Stearic Acid,
Triethanolamine, Vegetable Oil, Water.

Packed in a 150 ml tube

Hand Cream   Ref. BT 0387

COSHH Group A   pH 6.2

Almond Oil (Sweet), Avocado Oil, BHA, Cetearyl
Alcohol, Cocoa Butter, Dichlorobenzyl Alcohol, FD & C
Blue No. 1, FD & C Yellow No. 5, Glyceryl Stearate,
Lavender Oil, Methylchloroisothiazolinone, Mineral Oil,
Paraffin Wax, Propylene Glycol, Sodium Lauryl Sulphate,
Sodium Lactate, Water.

Available in 365 g jars

Massage Cream   Ref. BT 0425

COSHH Group A   pH 7.2

D & C Yellow No. 6, Dichlorobenzyl Alcohol, FD & C
Yellow No. 5, Glyceryl Stearate, Lavender Oil,

Methylchloroisothiazolinone, Mineral Oil, Oleyl Alcohol, Petrolatum, Polysorbate 20, Propylene Glycol, Propylparaben, Sodium Borate, Sorbitan Palmitate, Stearic Acid, Water.

Available in 365 g jars

Massage Oil   Ref. BT 0423

COSHH Group C

BHA, Caprylic/Capric Triglyceride, Grapeseed Oil, Mineral Oil.

Sizes available: 500 ml bottles

Body Contour Cream   Ref. BT 0434

COSHH Group A   pH 5.3

Aloe Vera Gel, Aluminium Magnesium Silicate, Cinnamon Oil, Dichlorobenzyl Alcohol, Ginger Oil, Methylchloroisothiazolinone, Methylsilanol Mannuronate, Plant Extracts, Polyglyceryl Methacrylate, Propylene Glycol, Sodium Lactate, Xanthan Gum, Zedoary Oil, Water.

Packed in a 150 ml tube

Body Conditioning Cream   Ref. BT 0436

COSHH Group A   pH 5.6

Caprylic/Capric Triglyceride, Cetearyl Alcohol, Cocoa Butter, Dichlorobenzyl Alcohol, Glyceryl Stearate, Lavender Oil, Methylchloroisothiazolinone, Methyl-paraben, Propylparaben, Propylene Glycol, Sodium PCA, Sodium Lactate, Xanthan Gum, Water.

Packed in a 150 ml tube

Hand and Body Lotion   Ref. BT 0389

COSHH Group A   pH 7.5

Aloe Vera Gel, Cocoa Butter, D & C Red No. 33,
Fragrance, Glyceryl Stearate, Glycerine, Lanolin Alcohol,
Methylchloroisothiazolinone, PPG-25 Laureth-25, Stearic
Acid, Triethanolamine, Xanthan Gum, Water.

Available in a 200 ml bottle

For the Shower and Bath

Shower Gel   Ref. BT 0480

COSHH Group E   pH 6.5

Lauryl Betaine, Lavender Oil, Methylchloroisothiazolin-
one, PEG-150 Distearate, PEG-6 Caprylic/Capric
Triglyceride, Rosemary Oil, Sodium Laureth Sulphate,
Tea Tree Oil, Water.

Packed in a 150 ml dispenser

Enriched Cream Bath   Ref. BT 0478

COSHH Group E   pH 6.6

Aloe Vera Gel, Chamomile Oil, Cocamide DEA, Lauryl
Betaine, Methylchloroisothiazolinone, PEG-6 Caprylic/
Capric Triglyceride, PEG-150 Distearate, PVA, Sodium
Laureth Sulphate, Water.

Available in a 200 ml bottle

Sun Protection

Sun Protect SPF 14   Ref. BT 0470

COSHH Group A   pH 6.5

Caprylic/Capric Triglyceride, Cocoa Butter, Dimethicone, Hydroxyoctacosanyl Hydroxystearate, Methoxy PEG-22/Dodecyl Glycol Copolymer, Methylparaben, Octyl Palmitate, PEG-45/Dodecyl Glycol Copolymer, Propylene Glycol, Propylparaben. Titanium Dioxide, Water.

Packed in a 100 ml tube

Sun Protect SPF 25+   Ref. BT 0472

COSHH Group A   pH 6.5

Caprylic/Capric Triglyceride, Cocoa Butter, Dimethicone, Hydroxyoctacosanyl Hydroxystearate, Methoxy PEG-22/Dodecyl Glycol Copolymer, Methylparaben, Octyl Palmitate, PEG-45/Dodecyl Glycol Copolymer, Propylene Glycol, Propylparaben, Titanium Dioxide, Water.
Packed in a 100 ml tube

Ampoules for Galvanic Therapy

Each ampoule contains the active ingredient in sterilised water, protected by methylchloroisothiazolinone and made ionisable by the presence of sodium citrate. All are available as 2 ml ampoules packed in boxes of ten.

Disincrustation   Ref. BT 0010

pH 9.2

Methylchloroisothiazolinone, Sodium Bicarbonate, Water.

Collagen Ref. BT 0010

pH 8.0

Carboxymethylcellulose, Collagen (Hydrolysed Vegetable Protein), Methylchloroisothiazolinone, Sodium Citrate, Water.

Aloe Vera Ref. BT 0010

pH 8.0

Aloe Vera Gel, Methylchloroisothiazolinone, Sodium Citrate, Water.

Ginseng Ref. BT 0010

pH 8.0

Extract of Ginseng, Methylchloroisothiazolinone, Sodium Citrate, Water.

Chamomile Ref. BT 0010

pH 8.0

Extract of Chamomile, Methylchloroisothiazolinone, Sodium Citrate, Water.

All Nature's Way galvanic products may be considered as non-hazardous under normal conditions of use, but due care should be exercised in handling the glass ampoules.

Aromatherapy

Aromatherapy Oils

Each Nature's Way aromatherapy oil is the pure unadulterated oil, available only in 14 ml amber glass bottles. The full list appears below:

Basil *Ocymum basilium*

Bergamot *Citrus bergamia*

Chamomile *Matricaria chamomilla*

Cypress *Cupressus sempervirens*

Eucalyptus *Eucalyptus globulus*

Fennel *Foeniculum vulgare*

Frankincense *Boswellia thurifera*

Geranium *Pelargonium odorantissimum*

Grapefruit *Citrus paradisi*

Juniper *Juniperus communis*

Lavender *Lavendula officinalis*

Lemon *Citrus limonum*

Lemongrass *Cymbopogon citratus*

Melissa *Melissa officinalis*

Peppermint *Mentha piperita*

Rosemary *Rosmarinus officinalis*

Sandalwood *Santalum album*

Tea Tree *Melaleuca alternifolia*

Ylang-Ylang *Cananga odorata*

Health and Safety Data — refer to COSHH Group D

Aromatherapy Carrier Oils

Each Nature's Way aromatherapy carrier oil is the pure unadulterated oil plus natural vitamin E to stabilise it against rancidity.

Avocado Oil   Available in 200 ml bottles.

Grapeseed Oil   Available in 200 ml and 500 ml bottles.

Sweet Almond Oil   Available in 200 ml and 500 ml bottles.

Wheat Germ Oil   Available in 200 ml bottles.

Health and Safety Data — all belong to COSHH Group D

Aromatherapy Pre-blended Oils for Body Massage

The pre-blended oils are the pure essential oils in a vegetable carrier oil, ready for use.

For Arthritis and Rheumatism   Ref. NWA 0240

COSHH Group D

Almond Oil (Sweet), plus Essential Oils of Eucalptus, Juniper, Rosemary and Vitamin E.

Available in 200 ml bottles

For Body Aches and Pains   Ref. NWA 0260

COSHH Group D

Grapeseed Oil, plus Essential Oils of Bergamot, Juniper, Lavender and Vitamin E Oil.

Available in 200 ml bottles

For Relaxing Bodily Stress   Ref. NWA 0280

COSHH Group D

Grapeseed Oil, plus Essential Oils of Chamomile, Juniper, Melissa and Vitamin E Oil.

Available in 200 ml bottles

For Cellulite and Fluid Retention   Ref. NWA 0250

COSHH Group D

Grapeseed Oil, plus Essential Oils of Fennel, Juniper, Rosemary and Vitamin E Oil.

Available in 200 ml bottles

For Stretch Marks   Ref. NWA 0270

COSHH Group D

Avocado Oil, plus Essential Oils of Frankincense, Lavender, Lemongrass and Vitamin E Oil.

Available in 200 ml bottles

Pre-blended Essential Oils for Facial Massage

For Oily and Problem Skin   Ref. NWA AO

COSHH Group D

Grapeseed Oil, plus Essential Oils of Bergamot, Lavender and Lemon and Vitamin E Oil.

Available in 100 ml bottles

For Dry and Sensitive Skin   Ref. NWA AO

COSHH Group D

Almond Oil (Sweet), plus Essential Oils of Chamomile, Sandalwood and Ylang-Ylang and Vitamin E Oil.

Available in 100 ml bottles

For Dry and Mature Skin   Ref. NWA AO

COSHH Group D

Almond Oil (Sweet) and Avocado Oil, plus Essential Oils of Geranium, Lavender, Sandalwood and Vitamin E Oil.

Available in 100 ml bottles

Nature's Way Aromatherapy Bases

Nature's Way aromatherapy bases are two unfragranced products, specially prepared for the user to add the essentials oils of his or her choice.

Facial Massage Cream   Ref. BT 0100

COSHH Group A pH 5.5

Almond Oil (Sweet), BHA, Cetearyl Alcohol, Cocoa Butter, Methylparaben, Polyvinylpyrrolidone, Propylene Glycol, Propylparaben, Sodium Lauryl Sulphate, Water.

Available in 100 g jars

Aromatherapy Mask Base   Ref. BT 0101

COSHH Group A   pH 7.3

Aloe Vera Gel, Carbomer, Dichlorobenzyl Alcohol, EDTA Disodium Salt, Glycerine, Methylchloroisothiazolinone, Polyvinylpyrrolidone, Stearyl Heptonate, Triethanolamine, Witch Hazel BPC, Water.

Available in 100 g jars

Chapter Ten

COSHH and Health and Safety

As you are probably aware, new health and safety regulations came into force on 1 January 1990. These are generally referred to as COSHH, which is an acronym for the "Control of Substances Hazardous to Health".

Briefly, the objective is to provide one set of regulations to cover the use of all substances hazardous to health. The regulations apply to substances that have been classified as Very Toxic, Toxic, Harmful, Corrosive or Irritant. They also cover materials with chronic or delayed effects such as carcinogens, mutagens and teratogens. In addition they cover materials in compound form, allergens and microbiological problems. Dust in high concentration is also considered a hazard.

Every employer is responsible for all his employees and, so far as is reasonably practicable, for other persons working in or visiting his or her premises.

Each employer must provide an assessment of the potential risk of any process or work activity which is liable to expose any employee to any substance hazardous to health. This assessment must be carried out by a competent person and be sufficient to identify and determine any potential risks.

It will be required to control exposure to such risks through the selection, use and maintenance of appropriate controls over materials, plant and processes. Only where these are not reasonably practicable will personal protection equipment be considered appropriate as a means of controlling exposure. It is also a requirement that employers maintain health surveillance records on their employees.

The principle of occupational hygiene practice upon which the regulations and codes of practice are based is mainly one of maintaining high standards of cleanliness and hygiene in the work place and ensuring that these standards are maintained by the workers. Fortunately, beauty clinics are usually models of cleanliness and hygiene.

All suppliers of materials or products to be used at a place of work, including of course hair and beauty salons, must advise the purchaser of any potential hazards. Bellitas Limited as suppliers of Nature's Way products, have a complete file of all risks that may be associated with the products. Copies are available on request; please quote the reference number, which is shown in chapter 9 against each product, to expedite a reply to your enquiry. Each Nature's Way product also carries a letter identifying the COSHH group to which it belongs (see chapter 9). In the present chapter you will find under each COSHH group letter, in generalised form, the health and safety data relevant to each group and applicable to all Nature's Way products.

By their nature, skin-care products can be considered as being very low risk, but because therapists are exposed to products for prolonged periods the following advice should be heeded.

Avoid prolonged contact with any product, especially through contaminated clothing. Aromatherapy oils, massage oils and skin toners may cause irritation if left on clothing in contact with the skin for prolonged periods. Undiluted products intended for use in the bath or shower or as wash-off cleansers may also cause irritation if prolonged skin contact occurs.

If any product enters the eye wash it thoroughly with cold water; if irritation persists seek medical attention. The list of ingredients and the product's pH will be useful information for the doctor.

None of Nature's Way products need be considered flammable.

Spillage is the worst potential hazard in any salon. The rule must be — if spilt, clean up immediately.

Product Safety Data

COSHH Group A. Emulsions: Cleansers, Moisturisers, Night Creams, Masks and Sun Protect Products.

Description Such products are an emulsion of oils, waxes, water and water-soluble ingredients and may contain colour, fragrance and preservatives.

Ingredients All ingredients are commonly used in cosmetic products and meet accepted standards of purity.

Hazard Such products are considered to be non-hazardous under normal conditions of use.

Flammability Non-inflammable.

First-Aid Procedures

Ingestion Drink milk or water.

Inhalation Not applicable.

Skin Contact Not applicable.

Eye Contact Wash well with water; if irritation persists seek medical advice.

Spillage Clean using absorbent material followed by wash with water to avoid slippery floors.

Handling No special precautions considered necessary.

Storage Store in a cool place away from direct sunlight.

Note: This information is furnished without warranty, either expressed or implied, but is believed to be accurate. However, no responsibility can be accepted for the consequences of misuse of this product.

Product Safety Data

COSHH Group B. Skin Toners.

Description These products are clear lotions, containing no more than 8% ethanol by weight, with water and water-soluble ingredients. They may contain colour, fragrance and preservatives.

Ingredients All ingredients are commonly used in cosmetic products and meet accepted standards of purity.

Hazard The product is not considered to be hazardous under normal conditions of use.

Flammability Non-inflammable.

Ethanol Content ≤8% w/w.

First-Aid Procedures

Ingestion Avoid; drink plenty of milk or water.

Inhalation Not considered hazardous.

Skin Contact Avoid prolonged contact with skin; if irritation persists seek medical advice.

Eye Contact Wash well with water; if irritation persists seek medical advice.

Spillage Clean contaminated area with lots of water; wash with detergent and water to avoid slippery floors.

Fire Contents are non-flammable.

Handling No special precautions considered necessary.

Storage Store in a cool place away from direct sunlight.

Note: This information is furnished without warranty, either expressed or implied, but is believed to be accurate. However, no responsibility can be accepted for the consequences of misuse of this product.

Product Safety Data

COSHH Group C. Massage and Aromatherapy Carrier Oils.

Description Such products are oily liquids.

Ingredients All ingredients meet accepted standards of purity for cosmetic use.

Hazard These products are considered to be non-hazardous under normal conditions of use.

Flammability Non-inflammable but will burn with noxious fumes.

First-Aid Procedures

Ingestion Non-hazardous but best avoided because of laxative effect.

Inhalation Not applicable.

Skin Contact Non-hazardous but avoid prolonged contact because of possible skin degreasing effect.

Eye Contact Wash well with water; if irritation persists seek medical advice.

Spillage Clean using absorbent material followed by wash with detergent and water to avoid slippery floors.

Storage Store in a cool place away from direct sunlight.

Handling No special precautions considered necessary.

Note: This information is furnished without warranty, either expressed or implied, but is believed to be accurate. However, no responsibility can be accepted for the consequences of misuse of this product.

Product Safety Data

COSHH Group D. Aromatherapy Essential Oils and Pre-blends.

Description Such products are oily liquids with a characteristic odour.

Ingredients All ingredients meet accepted standards of purity for cosmetic use.

Hazard These products are considered to be non-hazardous under normal conditions of use but all essential oils are reactive substances which should be used with due care and caution and according to instructions.

Flammability Non-inflammable but will burn with noxious fumes.

First-Aid Procedures

Ingestion Avoid; essential oils are for topical application only. If accidentally ingested drink plenty of milk or water and seek medical advice.

Inhalation Excessive exposure could lead to dizziness; seek fresh air and keep warm.

Skin Contact Non-hazardous but avoid excessive contact.

Eye Contact Wash well with water; if irritation persists seek medical advice.

Spillage Clean using absorbent material followed by wash with detergent and water to avoid slippery floors.

Storage Store in a cool place away from direct sunlight.

Handling No special precautions considered necessary.

Note: This information is furnished without warranty, either expressed or implied, but is believed to be accurate. However, no responsibility can be accepted for the consequences of misuse of this product.

Product Safety Data

COSHH Group E. Products for the Bath and Shower, Wash-off Cleansers and other products containing surfactants.

Description Such products are a mixture of cleaning and wetting agents with water and water-soluble ingredients and may contain conditioners, colour, fragrance and preservatives.

Ingredients All ingredients are commonly used in cosmetic products and meet accepted standards of purity.

Hazard These products are considered to be non-hazardous under normal conditions of use.

Flammability Non-inflammable.

First-Aid Procedures

Ingestion Drink milk or water.

Inhalation Not applicable.

Skin Contact Avoid prolonged contact with the concentrated product; if irritation occurs and persists seek medical advice.

Eye Contact Wash well with water, if irritation persists seek medical advice.

Spillage Clean using absorbent material followed by wash with water to avoid slippery floors.

Storage Store in a cool place away from direct sunlight.

Handling No special precautions considered necessary.

Note: This information is furnished without warranty, either expressed or implied, but is believed to be accurate. However, no responsibility can be accepted for the consequences of misuse of this product.

Bibliography

The numbered books are specifically referred to in the text.

1. Wilkinson, J.B., and Moore, R.J., eds. *Harry's Cosmeticology.* 7th edition. London: Longman, 1982.

2. Montagna, William, Parker, F., and Tosti, A. *Skin: Your Owner's Manual.* Rome: Antonio Delfino Editore, 1985.

3. Hylton, William H. *Rodale Herb Book.* Emmaus, Pennsylvania: Rodale Press, 1974.

4. Woodruff, John, and Jones, Elisabeth. *Aromatherapy and Cosmetic Science.* Weymouth, Dorset: Micelle Press. In preparation.

5. Gattefossé. *Aromathérapie,* 1928.

6. Valnet, J. *The Practice of Aromatherapy.* London: C.W. Daniel Company, 1982.

7. Tisserand, R. *The Essential Oil Safety Data Manual.* Hove, East Sussex: Tisserand Aromatherapy Institute, 1985.

8. Parry, E.J. *Parry's Cyclopedia of Perfumery.* 2 vols. London: J. & A. Churchill, 1925.

9. *Martindale: The Extra Pharmacopeia.* 29th edition. London: Pharmaceutical Press, 1989.

10. Nowak, G.A. *Cosmetic Preparations.* Translated by Philip Alexander. Vol. 1. Augsburg, Germany: H. Ziolkowsky, 1985.

11. Harry, Ralph. *The Principles and Practice of Modern Cosmetics, Vol. 2: Cosmetic Materials.* London: Leonard Hill, 1962.

12. Hunting, Anthony L.L. *Encyclopedia of Conditioning Rinse Ingredients.* London: Micelle Press, 1987.

Arnould-Taylor, W.E. *Aromatherapy for the Whole Person.* Cheltenham, Gloucestershire: Stanley Thornes, 1981.

Austermann, Ursula E.E. *A Compendium of Cosmetology and Aesthetics.* Cheltenham, Gloucestershire: Stanley Thornes, 1987.

Bembridge, R.A. *Beauty Therapy Science.* London: Longman, 1988.

Burton, J.L. *Essentials of Dermatology.* 2nd edition. London: Longman, 1985.

Gallant, Ann. *Principles and Techniques for the Beauty Specialist.* 2nd edition. Cheltenham, Gloucestershire: Stanley Thornes, 1980.

Gerson, Joel. *Standard Textbook for Professional Estheticians.* 2nd edition. New York: Milady Publishing, 1979.

Githa Goldberg, Audrey. *Care of the Skin.* 3rd edition. Oxford: Heinemann, 1988.

Haarmann & Reimer. *The H&R Book of Perfume.* Hamburg: R.Glöss, 1992.

Hagman, Anne, and Arnould-Taylor, W.E. *The Aestheticienne: Simple Theory and Practice.* Cheltenham, Gloucestershire: Stanley Thornes, 1981.

Howard, George, and Arnould-Taylor, W.E. *Principles and Practice of Perfumery and Cosmetics.* Cheltenham, Gloucestershire: Stanley Thornes, 1987.

Marks, Ronald. *The Sun and Your Skin.* London: Macdonald, 1988.

Middleton, A.W. *Cosmetic Science 1962.* London: Pergamon, 1963.

Simmons, John V. *Science and the Beauty Business, Vol. 1: The Science of Cosmetics.* London: Macmillan, 1989.

Simmons, John V. *Science and the Beauty Business, Vol. 2: The Beauty Salon and its Equipment.* London: Macmillan, 1989.

Tisserand, R. *The Art of Aromatherapy* London: C.W. Daniel Company, 1977.

Van Toller, Steve, and Dodd, George H., eds. *Perfumery: The Psychology and Biology of Fragrance.* London: Chapman & Hall, 1988.

Winyard, Gaynor. *A Guide for Health & Beauty Therapists, Vol. 1: Face, Hands and Feet.* London: Longman, 1990.

Index